WARD LOCK

FAMILY HEALTH GUIDE

EPILEPSY

ALICE HANSCOMB AND LIZ HUGHES

**IN ASSOCIATION WITH
THE NATIONAL SOCIETY FOR EPILEPSY**

WARD LOCK

Alice Hanscomb and Liz Hughes are recognized experts working as Information and Education Officers at the National Society for Epilepsy (NSE). They give lectures on the condition to professional and non-professional bodies as well as dealing with the many day-to-day issues raised by people with epilepsy. They write the educational literature to support the NSE National Helpline and are involved with international epilepsy education.

A WARD LOCK BOOK

First published in the UK 1995
by Ward Lock
Wellington House
125 Strand
London

WC2R OBB

A Cassell Imprint

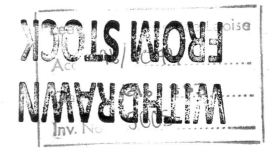

Distributed in the United States
by Sterling Publishing Co., Inc.
387 Park Avenue South, New York, NY 10016-8810

Distributed in Australia
by Capricorn Link (Australia) Pty Ltd
2/13 Carrington Road, Castle Hill, NSW 2154

A British Library Cataloguing in Publication Data block for this book may be obtained from the British Library.

ISBN 0 7063 7404 5
Designed by Lindsey Johns and typeset by The Design Revolution, Brighton
Printed and bound in Spain

Acknowledgements
The publishers would like to thank the National Society for Epilepsy for their help in producing this book, and for providing the photographs on pages 18, 19, 21, 22, 28, 37, 43 and 72. All other photographs are reproduced by permission of Life File. Cover photograph: Tony Stone Images.

Contents

Introduction

Epilepsy can happen to anyone at any time of life. People don't realize just how common it is: most of us have an idea of how common, say, diabetes is, but few are aware that similar numbers of people have epilepsy.

At least one in 200 members of the population have epilepsy at any one time, but most of these won't actually be experiencing seizures because they are controlled by the medication they take, so it is impossible to know if someone has epilepsy unless, of course, they tell you. Others may experience seizures many times every day or only once a week, once a month or perhaps just once a year. Some types of seizure are so subtle and are over so quickly that you would not even know they were happening; others may cause confused or strange behaviour. People usually think of someone with epilepsy as having a major convulsive seizure, but this is only one of many kinds.

Having epilepsy doesn't necessarily mean that someone can't do the things that they may like or want to do. People with epilepsy can work, drive, play sports, travel and have families just like anyone else.

The issues covered in this book are those raised by people with epilepsy and by their families who have contacted the National Society for Epilepsy's (NSE) National Helpline. The questions asked are many and varied and we have tried to include most of the topics on which we have received requests for information.

Alice Hanscomb
Liz Hughes

Note It is important to remember that some of the information given in this book does not apply to countries other than the UK. For example, the names of anti-epileptic drugs, and driving and employment regulations, are different in the USA and Australia.

Chapter one

So what is epilepsy?

Epilepsy is a physical condition in the same way as arthritis and blindness are. Whereas arthritis occurs in the joints, epilepsy occurs in the brain. A medical definition is 'repeated seizures of primary cerebral origin' which simply means that someone with epilepsy has a tendency to experience seizures which originate in the brain. Some people with diabetes may have seizures, but this isn't epilepsy because their seizures are a symptom of their body's inability to balance the sugar levels in the blood, rather than being a problem within the brain.

How the brain works

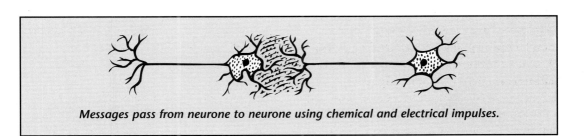

Messages pass from neurone to neurone using chemical and electrical impulses.

To understand this we need to look at how the brain works. The brain itself is made up of many millions of neurones (nerve cells), all of which are interconnected. Messages come into the brain from the rest of the body and the spinal cord, travelling along the nerve-fibres, and pass from neurone to neurone using chemical and electrical impulses. One of the brain's most important functions is to organize all these messages. To do so it uses two

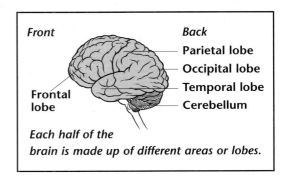

Front　　　　　　　*Back*
— **Parietal lobe**
— **Occipital lobe**
— **Temporal lobe**
Frontal lobe
— **Cerebellum**

Each half of the brain is made up of different areas or lobes.

7

So what is epilepsy?

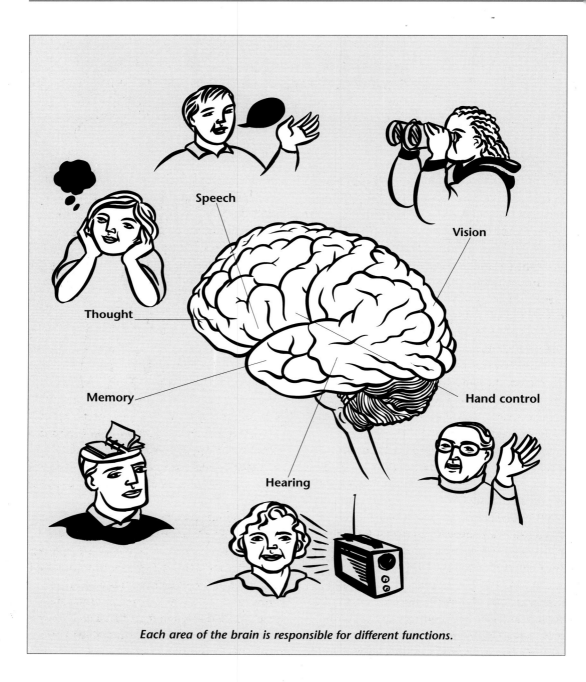

Each area of the brain is responsible for different functions.

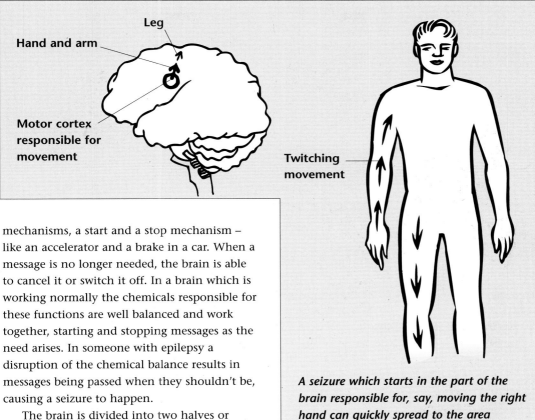

Hand and arm

Leg

Motor cortex
responsible for
movement

Twitching
movement

A seizure which starts in the part of the brain responsible for, say, moving the right hand can quickly spread to the area responsible for the right arm and leg.

mechanisms, a start and a stop mechanism – like an accelerator and a brake in a car. When a message is no longer needed, the brain is able to cancel it or switch it off. In a brain which is working normally the chemicals responsible for these functions are well balanced and work together, starting and stopping messages as the need arises. In someone with epilepsy a disruption of the chemical balance results in messages being passed when they shouldn't be, causing a seizure to happen.

The brain is divided into two halves or hemispheres (right and left), each made up of separate areas or lobes. Each area is responsible for different things.

When someone has a seizure, the way it looks like to an outsider and how it feels to the person experiencing it will depend on where in the brain this abnormal chemical activity begins and to where it spreads. So, for example, if the seizure starts in the part of the brain responsible for moving the right hand and spreads to the area responsible for moving the right arm and then the leg, the person experiencing the

seizure will first get a twitching in the right hand which will spread to involve the whole arm and then to cause twitching of the right leg as well. This will happen very quickly and could all be over in a matter of seconds or minutes. There are many different types of seizure and these will be covered in more detail in Chapter 3. There are also many different reasons why people have epilepsy.

So what is epilepsy?

Why do people have epilepsy?

There are many reasons why someone may develop epilepsy. Broadly speaking, these can be grouped together under three main headings: symptomatic, idiopathic and cryptogenic.

Types of epilepsy

- Symptomatic: a cause is found.
- Idiopathic: no cause is found but a genetic cause is suspected.
- Cryptogenic: no cause is found but a structural cause is suspected.

Symptomatic epilepsy

Epilepsy is known as symptomatic when a cause for the condition can actually be found. This could include head injury, scarring as a result of an infection of the brain, stroke or brain haemorrhage.

- Experiencing a **head injury**, perhaps as a result of a road traffic or sporting accident, does not always mean that the individual will develop epilepsy. If there has been bleeding inside the brain, or if there has been a long period of unconsciousness, there is a greater risk of seizures developing and the type of seizure will depend on where the damage occurred within the brain.
- **Infections of the brain** which could result in the individual developing epilepsy include meningitis, which affects the membranes covering the brain (the meninges); encephalitis, a virus affecting the brain tissues; and infections of the brain tissue such as brain abscesses. The chance of developing seizures as a result of these infections is lessened if they are diagnosed early and treatment is started quickly.
- **Brain tumours**, both malignant and benign, have the potential to cause epileptic seizures.
- Sometimes there are **structural abnormalities** if the brain of the unborn child did not develop properly while it was still in the mother's womb. There may also have been damage caused during birth: for example, if the delivery was long and complicated, the baby may have been deprived of oxygen. This is still quite a common cause of epilepsy in some developing countries because of poor obstetric care, but it is becoming far less common in the West.
- Some people may be born with a **birth mark on their brain** in the same way that others are born with birth marks on the skin and this may cause them to have seizures.

Idiopathic epilepsy

In up to 50 per cent of people diagnosed as having epilepsy no cause can be found, and their condition is known as idiopathic. It is thought that in some of these the tendency to experience seizures is inherited – that is, there is a genetic cause. In fact each one of us has such a tendency and we would all experience seizures under certain circumstances. Everyone has a particular level of resistance to them, however, and this is called a seizure threshold. In some people the seizure threshold may be especially high, while in others it may be very low, and it is this second group who may experience seizures spontaneously, for no apparent cause. It is thought that the seizure threshold too is inherited; however, it is not as straightforward as it may seem, so let's look at this in more detail.

Cryptogenic epilepsy

Cryptogenic epilepsy is another type in which no cause can be found, but unlike idiopathic epilepsy it is not thought to have developed for any genetic reason; instead there is an undiscovered physical cause which is yet to be found. It is possible that this physical cause is so small that the tests currently available are not yet sophisticated enough to pinpoint it. With increasing knowledge and improved diagnostic techniques, such as magnetic resonance imaging (see page 21), it is thought that the numbers within this group will begin to diminish and that it will be possible to discover causes of epilepsy for more and more people.

Can epilepsy be inherited?

The simple answer to this question is no. However, some people may have inherited a trait which makes them more likely to develop epilepsy. For example, if a mother has epilepsy because she has a low seizure threshold, a child of hers may inherit that low seizure threshold. But if the child's father has a high seizure threshold, the child, having inherited from both parents, may not have a seizure threshold low enough to cause him or her to develop epilepsy.

Sometimes it also takes an outside factor to trigger the start of epilepsy. Someone may have an inherited low resistance to seizures but may not develop them unless they go through a particularly stressful time in their life, for example, or perhaps suffer a mild head injury which lowers their resistance even further. It is only then that the epilepsy starts. It must be remembered that if the sole cause of the epilepsy is a head injury (for example, from a road traffic accident), the condition will not be inherited – just as you cannot inherit a broken leg.

Sometimes epilepsy can be seen to affect certain families and this could imply that there is a low seizure threshold common to the members of these families. It could, of course, be coincidental, taking into consideration how common the condition is.

It is also possible, although rare, for a child to inherit a genetic disease, a symptom of which may be epilepsy. Examples include tuberous sclerosis or neurofibromatosis.

Therefore it can be said that it is not epilepsy which is inherited; it is either a low seizure threshold or a genetic disease or syndrome which may result in seizures.

So what is epilepsy?

When is the most common time of life to develop epilepsy?

The age group in which epilepsy most commonly makes a first appearance is the under-20s, and there are many reasons for this. Very occasionally seizures may even begin while the unborn child is still in the mother's womb and will continue after the baby is born. Some people, as we have seen, are born with a low seizure threshold and this alone may cause them to have seizures; others are born with an existing physical cause for their seizures. It is also true that children and young people are more at risk of suffering brain damage in childhood accidents or by infections which may in turn lead to seizures, as their skulls and brains are not yet fully developed.

The second most common age group in which epilepsy develops is the over-60s. Older people become more susceptible to stroke and other cardio-vascular problems, and because the brain may be damaged as a result of any of these they may go on to develop epilepsy. It is recognized that the condition is growing more and more common in the older age group, partly because people are generally living longer. It is important that older people are diagnosed and treated as a younger person would be and that seizures do not go unidentified or ignored. Developing epilepsy at this time of life may have many implications: the increased risk of injury and the interaction between different forms of drug treatment are just two examples.

Epilepsy syndromes

Some children may develop what is known as an epilepsy syndrome, one of the symptoms of which is seizures. The subject of epilepsy syndromes is a highly complicated one. Children with particular syndromes show signs of slow development and learning difficulties from an early age, and the results from an electro-encephalogram (EEG) – see Chapter two – and the seizure type will help the doctor diagnose the type of syndrome the child may have. Epilepsy syndromes are rare and include, among others, Lennox-Gastaut, Landau Kleffner and West syndrome. The child's doctor will be able to provide the parent with more information about the particular type of syndrome.

Between the ages of 20 and 60 it is less usual to develop epilepsy than at other times, but some of the common causes within this age group include tumours, head injuries (resulting from road traffic, sporting or work accidents) or excessive alcohol or drug abuse.

However, it should be remembered that many adults who experience epilepsy for the first time at this period of their life may have idiopathic epilepsy, in which their seizures occur out of the blue without any apparent cause or damage to the brain.

Will the epilepsy ever go away?

In the same way as epilepsy can start at any age and without any apparent cause, some people find that their epilepsy simply goes away. This is called spontaneous remission, and it occurs most commonly in children who just grow out of their epilepsy, often on reaching puberty. Children with a syndrome known as benign Rolandic epilepsy always grow out of their epilepsy, usually by the age of 15 or 16, after which they will no longer have seizures.

It is often impossible for doctors to tell whether or not someone's epilepsy will simply go away (or remiss). Very often it is a matter of wait and see. However, it is always important to carry on taking anti-epileptic medication while there is a risk of having seizures.

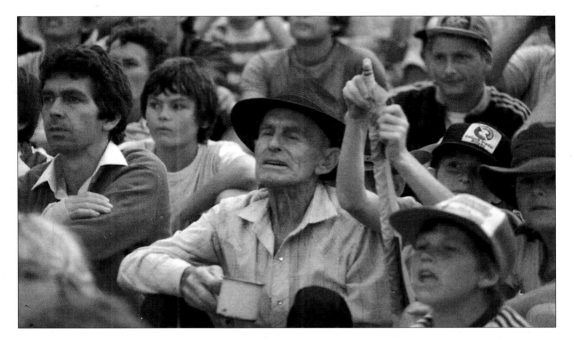

Anyone can develop epilepsy at any time of their life.

Chapter two

How does the doctor know it's epilepsy?

Having established what epilepsy is, and that anyone can develop the condition at any time of life, how is the diagnosis actually made? The diagnostic process, which may take some weeks or months, will usually start with the family doctor. When someone goes to their doctor worried because something has happened to them – for example, they experienced something they cannot explain or they blacked out – they will be sitting in front of him or her without showing any visible symptoms. The only thing the doctor will have to go on is what the patient tells him or her. It is therefore very helpful for the doctor if the individual brings someone with them who was there when the 'episode' occurred so that this second individual can describe to the doctor what they saw.

What is the diagnosis of epilepsy actually based upon?

There are a number of tests which can be carried out that will help to pinpoint the possible cause of what has happened. Some tests are done to rule out the more obvious causes for the episode or episodes, such as blood tests and electrocardiograms (ECGs), which are discussed in more depth below. These being clear (that is, showing no sign of abnormality), the family doctor is likely to refer the person to a specialist for a diagnosis. Children will see a consultant paediatrician or paediatric neurologist, adults should see a consultant neurologist and elderly people may be referred to a geriatrician specializing in neurology. Not all neurologists specialize in epilepsy and those who do will often see people who have already been diagnosed but are experiencing further problems.

It is at this point that further tests, such as EEGs and brain scans, may be carried out to help the specialist make an accurate diagnosis. But as most people will have either normal or inconclusive results back from these tests, what is a diagnosis of epilepsy actually based upon? The most important information for the specialist to have, like the family doctor, is that given by the person in the form of a description of what they have experienced, together with their medical history. However, the person may not have been conscious during the episodes or may not remember all of what happened, so if someone else was present at the time, their account of what happened is obviously vitally important. It is upon this description that the diagnosis is based. The results of the tests may support it, but the diagnosis of epilepsy rests upon what actually happened and under what circumstances.

If only one or two seizures or episodes have occurred, the doctor may be reluctant or slow to make any kind of diagnosis. In fact some people may never experience more than just one or two seizures, so this would not necessarily warrant a diagnosis of epilepsy unless the test results were totally conclusive. But also, going by so few occurrences, the doctor may not have all the information he or she needs and may advise that the best thing to do is to wait to see if anything else happens before making a diagnosis or starting the person on treatment. The doctor is also very aware that a diagnosis of epilepsy has important consequences for the person concerned: for instance, it could affect their driving licence, and it may affect the work that they do. Therefore the diagnosis is not made lightly.

This can be an extremely worrying and frustrating time if there is no explanation for the episodes, no treatment has been prescribed and nobody knows if they will occur again.

Seeing the consultant or specialist

It can take some time to get to see a consultant. It is a recognized fact that there are not enough neurologists in the UK and that, although the numbers are slowly increasing, the waiting lists can be long. (Because of this some people may see a registrar rather than a consultant, and it is important to be aware that registrars, like consultants, are very highly trained.) It is obviously advisable to arrive at the hospital in plenty of time for the appointment, but bear in mind that clinics may run late, so it is a good idea to be prepared for a long wait. Having someone with you and taking a good book to read will help pass the time.

The consultant, just like the family doctor, will need the answers to a number of questions (see the box on page 16) and it helps to give some thought to these before you see him or her.

Obviously answers to some of these questions can be given only by someone who was there at the time and saw what happened. It must be stressed, however, that no matter how qualified observers feel they are to make a judgement about what they witnessed, they must not do so. An accurate account of what happened is vital: a comment like, 'It was a seizure. I know it was, I've seen them before,' is not only unhelpful but could also bias the outcome of the diagnosis.

There are many reasons why people may lose consciousness, convulse, pass out or experience odd sensations. These include panic attacks, migraine, temper tantrums, faints, stroke or heart disease. Symptoms of these other conditions are occasionally mistaken for epileptic seizures and this is when a mis-diagnosis can be made (see page 24 for more details). The answers to the questions the

How does the doctor know it's epilepsy?

Examples of questions a consultant may ask

- Did the episodes occur out of the blue, or was there any warning immediately before they happened? (If there was a warning, a detailed description of this will be asked for.)
- How were you before the episodes occurred? Were you tired, hungry, thirsty, hot or very emotional? Were you very anxious or under extreme stress at the time?
- Did you feel unwell before the events – did you feel sick, dizzy, faint or breathless, or have chest pains or palpitations? If so, how long before the episodes occurred did you experience any of these?
- What were you doing when the episodes occurred?
- What actually happened to you before, during and after each episode?
- How long did each episode last?
- Can you remember what happened during the episodes? If you can't, what was the first thing you remembered afterwards?
- How did you feel after each episode was over? Did you experience any problems with your memory or feeling in any part of your body or have any muscle weakness or ache?
- Had you been to see a doctor before these occurred and had you been prescribed any medication?
- How often have the episodes occurred and have they affected you in exactly the same way each time? If not, each episode will need to be described in detail.
- Have you ever abused drugs or alcohol and if so has this been recently?
- Were there any birth complications when you were born?
- Have you ever had any kind of head injury?
- Did you ever experience any convulsions with a high temperature when you were young?
- Has anyone else in your family ever experienced anything like this or ever been diagnosed as having epilepsy?

doctor may ask, the blood test and ECG will help to rule out these other physical conditions, but where there is doubt the doctor may need more evidence to go on so will delay making a diagnosis.

Since the doctor is so reliant on the information provided to make an accurate diagnosis, it is important to get that information right. As the consultant's appointment may be some time after the episode has occurred, it is useful for all concerned if detailed notes are made soon after the episode, so that information is not forgotten. The notes can then be taken into the consultation, and it is also often very helpful to take a pen and paper to make notes of what is said as the detail of the conversation can easily be forgotten afterwards. Having looked at the questions the consultant may ask, let us consider questions that you could ask the consultant.

Examples of questions to ask the consultant

- What do you think I experienced?
- What tests will you be putting me forward for and why?
- Should I continue to drive? If not do I need to inform the DVLA?
- Will you be starting me on any treatment? If so, what sort and how will this help?
- How likely is it that this will happen again?
- What has caused this to happen?

- Are you going to make a formal diagnosis now? If so, what?
- Is there anything either I or my family can do to help the situation?
- What should my family or anyone with me do if this happens again?
- Where can I go to get further information about what you have told me?
- How often do I need to come back for appointments with you?
- Where do we go from here?

Some people find it helpful to write down the answers to these questions so that nothing is forgotten. Others complain that the consultant does not answer their questions, and mostly this will be because he or she does not have all the answers. For example, very often the consultant will not be able to say at this stage whether the episode will happen again or may not be able to give a reason why it has happened.

Let us look at why the various tests are done and what is involved.

Diagnostic tests

Blood tests

A small sample of blood will be taken and analysed to find out if the liver, kidneys and other bodily organs are working as they should and that the person is in good health generally. If the blood test reveals a problem with any of the organs in the body, the cause is then pinpointed and suitable treatment can be started. For most people, however, the results of this initial blood test will be normal.

Electrocardiogram (ECG)

The ECG is not a standard diagnostic test and is carried out in only a few select cases. Its purpose is to show how the heart is working. An ECG will reveal if some sort of heart problem is responsible for what the person has experienced. Again, most people will have a clean bill of health after this test too.

Having ruled out problems originating in the body, the doctor will request tests on the remaining and most complicated organ – the

How does the doctor know it's epilepsy?

brain. This is commonly when the person is referred to a consultant neurologist.

Electroencephalogram (EEG)

An EEG is the next standard test to be done. Its purpose is to make a recording of the brain's activity or brain waves, which it does by picking up the tiny electrical signals given off by the communicating nerve cells (neurones). This recording will show if the neurones in the brain are 'firing' or communicating in a normal regular manner, or whether some are firing in an unusual irregular way. Most people given this test (including those who then go on to have a diagnosis of epilepsy made) will have a normal EEG reading because their neurones

were functioning normally during the test. In fact 20 per cent of people with epilepsy have a normal EEG because the only time when the neurones work abnormally is during a seizure, and unless they have a seizure while the test is being done, the EEG recording will be normal.

In some people, however, the EEG will pick up a continuous irregularity even when the person isn't having seizures.

If the person has a seizure during the EEG (though this is quite unlikely unless they are very frequent), and if the seizure is epileptic in origin, the EEG will record it and may suggest

EEG is a painless diagnostic test which usually takes about 20–30 minutes.

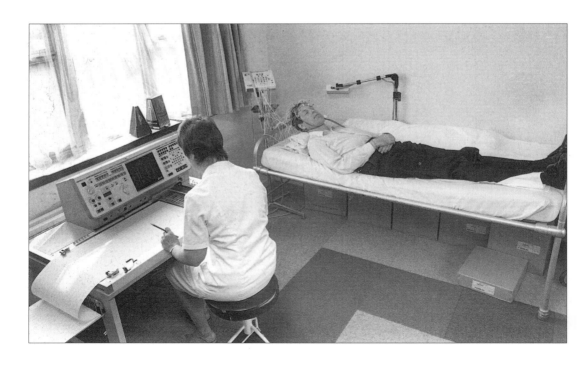

in which area of the brain the seizure activity started and which parts of the brain were affected. It may also show which type of seizure has occurred, which may help the doctor decide the kind of treatment required. Absence seizures (see page 30), for instance, have a very distinctive EEG pattern. Less conclusive EEG results may simply reveal that the person's brain wave pattern does not match the 'average'. This will be shown in at least 50 per cent of the general population. We are all unique in one way or other and some people will show a certain 'irregularity' in the way their brain cells communicate. This 'irregularity' of brain wave pattern can also be seen in some people who have migraines.

Having an abnormal EEG test result, therefore, does not automatically mean that the person has epilepsy. But neither does a normal test result mean that someone does *not* have epilepsy. This is a very common point of confusion. 'Why does my doctor think I have epilepsy when my EEG test results are normal?' is a question frequently asked on the National Society for Epilepsy's national helpline. Doctors, therefore, use the results as just one piece of evidence in their search for a diagnosis.

Absences are often mistaken for day-dreaming. EEG recordings can clearly show the distinctive changes in brain wave patterns.

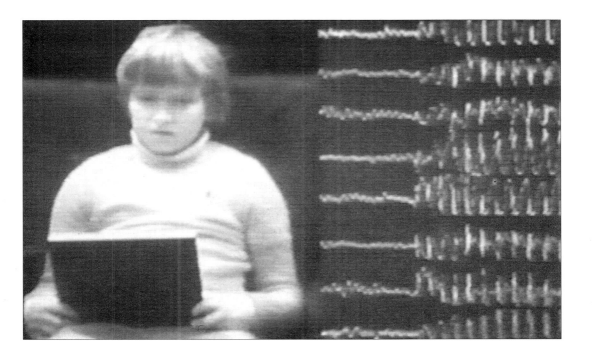

How does the doctor know it's epilepsy?

Nevertheless, the EEG test is an important one that everyone who is suspected of having epilepsy should undergo.

EEGs are used in a number of ways. Standardly, the test will last for 20–30 minutes, though longer tests may be requested. Sometimes a person may be asked to go without sleep for a night before having their EEG test so that they are drowsy or so that they may sleep during the test. This may help give a clearer test result as occasionally abnormal readings show up more readily when someone is tired or asleep.

What does having an EEG actually involve?

To record the tiny electrical impulses in the brain about 20 small, flat, metallic pads are stuck to the scalp with a kind of adhesive jelly. Each pad is attached to a wire which goes into the EEG machine. This in turn produces a readout showing a series of spiky wavy lines. The person is asked to lie very still on a couch or sit in a comfortable chair for the 20 or 30 minutes it takes to do the test. They will be asked to open and close their eyes regularly and will usually be asked to breathe deeply for a few minutes at some point during the test. They may also be asked to look at a flashing light for a few seconds at a time to find out whether the readout changes in response to certain frequencies of flashing light. The procedure is painless. When the test has been completed, the pads are carefully removed. The glue used to stick the pads on to the scalp is harmless but can be difficult to remove from the hair and several washes may be necessary to get rid of it

completely. It is then a matter of going back to the doctor for the results.

EEG ambulatory monitoring

As its name suggests, EEG ambulatory monitoring is a 'mobile EEG' test, enabling the person to be monitored at home. A small recording device rather like a personal stereo is worn on a belt around the waist. The small EEG pads are stuck firmly to the scalp and then well hidden under the hair. The wires connecting the pads to the recording box are then concealed under the clothes. The ambulatory monitor can be worn during most normal day-to-day activities, but must not come into contact with water, so showers and hair washes are not allowed. This test can be continued for many days with visits to the EEG technician necessary every 24 hours to change the tape and batteries. EEG ambulatory monitoring is usually available from specialist centres or clinics.

Video telemetry

Video telemetry is used for a number of different reasons: when diagnosis is proving difficult, for identifying seizure type or to find out whether someone is suitable for surgical treatment. This test involves both EEG and video recordings being made at the same time. As with ambulatory monitoring, video telemetry is done to try to record a seizure, so may need to be carried out over a number of days. The EEG pads are attached to the scalp as before and the person is usually able to move freely around the telemetry room within view of the video camera. Telemetry rooms are

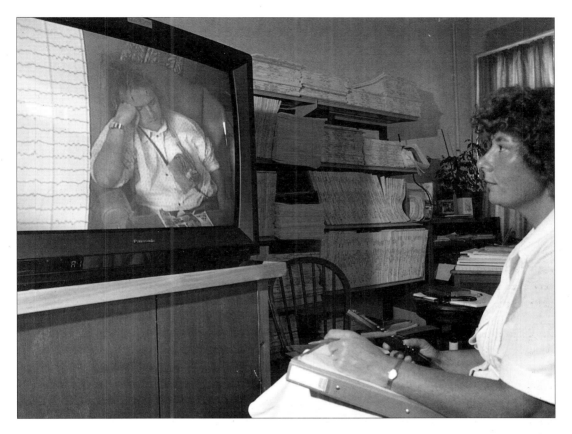

If someone has a seizure while a video telemetry recording is being carried out, there is video and EEG evidence of what happened.

usually well equipped with a comfortable chair, bed, television and chairs for visitors.

Brain scans

There are a number of different scans which include computerized tomography (CT or CAT) scans, magnetic resonance imaging (MR or MRI) and positron emission tomography (PET). These scans are carried out to discover if someone has symptomatic epilepsy: that is, if there is a structural cause for their seizures.

Computerized tomography (CT or CAT) scans use computerized X-ray techniques and will reveal any very obvious structural abnormality or damage which may be present.

Magnetic resonance imaging (MRI) does not work with active substances or X-rays. It uses harmless magnetic fields and radio

21

How does the doctor know it's epilepsy?

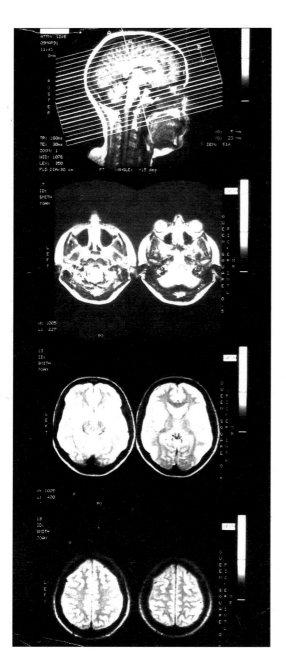

waves to form an image of the structure of the brain. The major difference between this and the CT scan is in the degree of detail it provides. MRI can reveal far smaller structural abnormalities than the CT scan and so is preferred by many doctors. This advanced ability to identify tiny lesions and points of scarring in the brain make it a vital part of the series of tests carried out to find out if someone is suitable for brain surgery. (This is discussed in Chapter four.) Not everyone needs to have an MR scan as it is used only if a structural cause for seizures is suspected.

Positron emission tomography (PET) reveals how the brain functions: for example, the way in which blood flows around it. To enable this to be monitored an active substance is injected into the bloodstream which can be 'seen' by the scanner. This in turn is then able to show the blood flow around different parts of the brain. The resulting 'picture' will reveal any areas of the brain which are not being fed by the bloodstream as well as the other areas are. It can also show blood flow from moment to moment, so highlighting which parts of the brain are most active. PET scans are used only in a very few people, usually solely for research purposes, and even then only infrequently because of the hazard of radiation.

These pictures produced by MRI show images of the brain taken from different levels through the head. The detailed structures of the brain are clearly shown.

What is involved in having a brain scan?

The procedure for having a scan will depend on the type. Most will involve lying on a cushioned flat surface which moves very slowly into a large round tunnel open at both ends. The person is asked to lie very still for between 5 and 15 minutes at a time while the 'pictures' of the brain are being taken. The scan process is likely to last about an hour in total. If someone who is going for a scan suffers with claustrophobia, they should tell the hospital this before they go and they may be given a light sedative to ease any anxiety during the scan.

MRI Before having an MR scan the person is usually given an information sheet to make sure that they come prepared and so that they know what to expect. Because MRI uses magnetic fields, there are certain items which cannot be worn or carried during the scan either by the patient or by anyone who comes into the scanning area with them: watches, metallic hair grips and credit cards, for instance. Certain people may not be able to have an MR scan because of some other medical condition – for example, if they have a pacemaker, or if they are in their first trimester of pregnancy – but the doctor will always

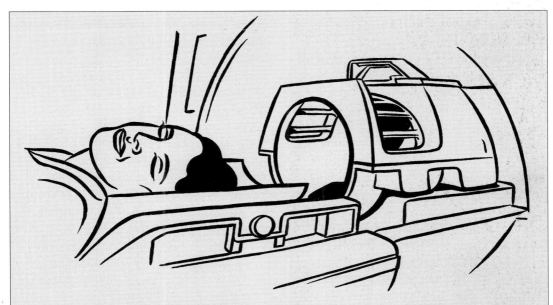

Someone having an MR scan will be asked to lie down on a cushioned surface which moves slowly inside the scanner. They will be asked to lie as still as possible while the 'pictures' of the brain are being taken.

How does the doctor know it's epilepsy?

advise on the suitability of each test for which he or she refers the person. MR scanners are renowned for producing a loud knocking sound while they are working and some people find this unnerving. But the staff will do all they can to make the experience as pleasant as possible and will make sure that the person is comfortable at each stage of the procedure.

PET The major difference between a PET scan and other forms is that this technique involves the injection of a radio-active substance which the scan can trace as it enters the brain. The injection is usually given in the arm and the needle needs to remain in place until the scan is over, which can make the arm quite sore afterwards.

What epilepsy is not

Febrile convulsions

Febrile convulsions are convulsive attacks which occur in young children, usually under the age of five years, when there is a sudden rise in their body temperature – for instance, at the beginning of a fever. These attacks affect many children and are the natural response of the immature brain to a sudden temperature increase. It is not the temperature which is reached but the speed at which it rises which is important. As the child gets older and the brain develops, it will no longer respond in this way.

It is important, as with any convulsive attack, that a febrile convulsion does not continue for too long, because a prolonged attack results in a loss of oxygen to the brain and this in turn could cause brain damage. Try to lower the body temperature as quickly as possible, perhaps by sponging the child down with cool water and encouraging him or her to drink cool fluids. It is important to report any attack to the family doctor and to make sure you know what to do should one happen again. Some children who experience febrile convulsions may go on to develop epilepsy, but

this would not be connected with a febrile convulsion early in life unless it had been prolonged and damage had occurred as a result. It is also true to say that some children may experience both febrile convulsions and epileptic seizures during the same period of their life.

Non-epileptic attacks

The subject of non-epileptic attacks is a very complicated one. When someone is said to have a non-epileptic attack disorder (NEAD), it means that although the seizures look very much like epileptic ones, they are not caused by epilepsy. In the past they may have been referred to as pseudo-seizures, but this term is being used less and less as our knowledge of the complexity of this disorder increases. There are many underlying reasons for non-epileptic attacks in the same way that there are a number of different causes of epilepsy.

Some people actually mimic epileptic seizures in an attempt to control certain circumstances or people. People with a learning disability who have seen others having seizures

Causes of non-epileptic attacks

Non-epileptic attacks can have either a physical or psychological cause.
- **Physical causes** include hypoglycaemia (low blood sugar) and faints.
- **Psychological causes** include panic attacks, delayed response to extreme stress and emotional cut-off.

receiving sympathy and help may also want to receive similar attention and so copy what they have seen. These non-epileptic seizures may occur in people with a history of epilepsy. Most people with non-epileptic attacks, however, do not 'put them on' but experience the attacks in the same way as people with epilepsy experience theirs – suddenly and unpredictably.

Panic attacks can look very similar to epileptic seizures and can be very frightening for the person experiencing them. They initially occur in response to a fearful situation but over time may happen independently of the situation. During a panic attack the person may hyperventilate, have palpitations, feel light-headed, have muscular spasms and even become unconscious.

Attacks which happen as a delayed response to extreme stress can occur as part of post traumatic stress disorder or in flashbacks to a stressful situation. The attack may begin with overbreathing, followed by screaming or crying which cannot be controlled. The person may

not remember what has happened once the attack is over.

Some people will experience an attack when they are unable to cope with the emotional demands or stress of a situation, and this is called emotional cut-off. Initially the attacks will occur only as a response to the specific stressful situation, but after a while they may occur during non-stressful situations as well. During the attack the person collapses and lies

How do you help someone having a non-epileptic attack?

Regardless of a seizure's cause – and, of course, in most cases it is impossible to tell what sort of attack it is – you should use your common sense and make the person having the attack as safe as possible. If the person is having a non-convulsive non-epileptic attack, simply keep them away from danger and stay with them until the attack is over. If someone is convulsing, make sure that you put something soft under the head, and once the attack has finished put them on their side in the recovery position (see page 29). As with all seizures there should be minimal fuss made and things should carry on as normal. Simply check that the person is all right and let them recover in their own time.

25

unconscious, unresponsive for a few minutes.

Because non-epileptic attacks are not caused by epilepsy, anti-epileptic drug treatment will not be effective. Anti-epileptic drugs treat epilepsy, not non-epileptic attacks. However, there are some people who will experience both non-epileptic attacks and epileptic seizures, and therefore will be prescribed anti-epileptic medication to control the epilepsy. If non-epileptic attacks are found to have a psychological cause, the individual will need to be referred to a psychologist or psychiatrist for treatment.

As previously stated, a diagnosis of epilepsy is not made lightly, and neither is a diagnosis of non-epileptic attack disorder.

Coming to terms with a diagnosis of epilepsy

Many people find a diagnosis of epilepsy particularly difficult to believe if the tests they have had show either inconclusive results or, more commonly, results that are clear. Being given the reasons for this will obviously help, but it can still be a time of great anxiety for the person concerned as well as for the whole family. People will react to the diagnosis in different ways. Many are very shocked to hear that they have epilepsy and will show signs of being 'in shock' for some time after the diagnosis has been made. Others may feel very relieved because they now know what their 'problem' is and treatment can at last be started. Some people will react very angrily, because being diagnosed as having epilepsy will have such a major impact on their lifestyle or employment. Most people will probably feel a bit of all these things and it is only natural for someone to be upset by the diagnosis for some time afterwards.

Because it can be an extremely difficult time for all concerned it is important to be able to talk over the situation with someone who understands what you are going through and what is involved in the process of diagnosis. Family doctors, epilepsy specialist nurses, counsellors and people on epilepsy helplines can provide this understanding and help. They may also be able to recommend other sources of help or useful information such as a contact at a local self-help group.

Now that we have looked at how a diagnosis of epilepsy is made, the next chapter will examine the many different types of epileptic seizure.

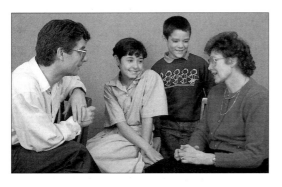

Being able to talk to someone about how you feel is always very helpful.

Chapter three

Types of epileptic seizure

The International Classification of Seizures is the most commonly used way of categorizing epileptic seizures (see the diagram on page 32). It does this according to the EEG recording and by what actually happens during the attack, but it doesn't take into account the cause of the seizures. It was suggested by the International League Against Epilepsy (ILAE), an international organization of professionals in different countries who specialize in the condition. It is this classification we are using here.

We will now look at the different types of seizure and what practical help can be given.

Types of seizure

The type of seizure someone experiences will depend on which part of the brain is being affected by seizure activity.

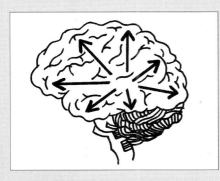

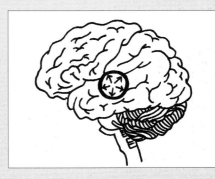

● In a **generalized seizure** the whole of the brain is affected.

● In a **partial or focal seizure** only a part of the brain is affected.

Types of epileptic seizure

Generalized seizures

During a generalized seizure the person is unconscious and totally unaware of what is happening. They will have no memory of it once it is over.

Tonic clonic seizure (previously known as grand mal)

When people think of an epileptic seizure, tonic clonic is the type that usually comes to mind. The term tonic clonic actually means stiffening and jerking, and this is exactly what happens when someone has a seizure of this kind. First, all the muscles in the body tighten and then go on to relax and tighten rhythmically and in quick succession, causing the person to convulse. The seizure may begin with a loud cry, which is caused by any air in the lungs being forced out through the voice box. Even though it may sound as if the person is in pain, they are not. They are unconscious and therefore unaware that they have even made the sound. During the convulsions a great deal of excess saliva can be produced, and if this is forced through tightly shut teeth it will result in the characteristic 'foaming at the mouth'. The person's breathing can sound very laboured during the seizure, but will quickly return to normal once the seizure is over. It is also possible that they may be incontinent during the seizure.

Having come out of a tonic clonic seizure, people are often confused, with no knowledge of what has happened or where they are, and they may have a bad headache. Because the muscles have all been working so hard during

the seizure, the person experiencing the attack may be very tired and may need to sleep for some time. They may also feel muscular aches and pains for even days afterwards.

How can I help?
The most important thing to do if someone has a tonic clonic seizure is to remain calm. It can be quite frightening to watch, but remember that the person experiencing the seizure is unconscious and will know nothing of what is going on, so feels no pain.

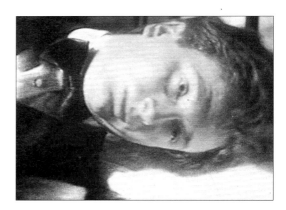

If someone has a tonic clonic seizure it can be frightening to watch, but it is important to keep calm. Put something soft under their head to prevent injury.

During the seizure:
● **Do** put something soft under the person's head, such as a rolled-up coat or cardigan, to prevent them from hurting themselves. If there

is nothing like this available, cup your hands under their head.

● **Do**, if you can, move away any object against which the person could hurt

themselves. If this is not possible, put something soft between the object and the person to prevent bruising. Move them only if they are in any danger.

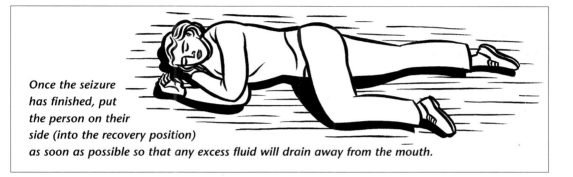

Once the seizure has finished, put the person on their side (into the recovery position) as soon as possible so that any excess fluid will drain away from the mouth.

Things not to do

● **Do not** move the person unless they are in a dangerous position – for example, at the top of a flight of stairs, in the road or near a fire or hot radiator.
● **Do not** put anything in the person's mouth.
● **Do not** give them anything to eat or drink until they have fully regained consciousness.
● **Do not** try to restrain the person.

Once the convulsions have stopped and the seizure has finished:
● **Do** put the person on to their side (into the recovery position) as soon as possible, so that any excess fluid will drain away.

● **Do** wipe away any excess saliva and, if the person still isn't breathing properly once the seizure has stopped, check that nothing is blocking their throat such as dentures or food.
● **Do** all that you can to minimize the embarrassment of the person when they come round. Try to keep others from gathering around and quietly reassure the person that they are OK, reminding them where they are as they may not be aware of their surroundings. If they have been incontinent, clear away any mess as quickly as you can.

Tonic seizure
In a tonic seizure consciousness is lost and there is a sudden stiffening of the person's whole body as the muscles tighten. If standing when the seizure occurs, the person will fall over. Unlike in a tonic clonic seizure there are no convulsions and recovery is quick.

Types of epileptic seizure

Atonic seizure

Sometimes known as a drop attack, the atonic seizure is the opposite of the tonic. In a tonic seizure the body is rigid; in an atonic seizure the person's body suddenly loses all muscle tone and goes floppy like a puppet which has had its strings cut and collapses to the floor. There are no convulsions and the person is unconscious throughout the brief attack.

How can I help?

In both tonic and atonic seizures, because the person may fall heavily to the floor, there are often injuries which may need medical attention. Stay with the person until they are ready to continue with what they were doing or, if there has been an injury because of the heavy fall, call for medical assistance.

Absence seizure (previously known as petit mal)

An absence is a rare form of seizure which can occur at any age but is most commonly seen in childhood or adolescence when it can easily be mistaken for day-dreaming. The person will look blank and stare into space for a few seconds, completely oblivious as to what is going on around them: not hearing, seeing or responding to anything while the seizure is in progress. When someone experiences an absence, they are unconscious for sometimes just a few seconds, which causes them to stop what they are doing. When they regain consciousness, they will carry on with whatever they were doing before the seizure occurred, often unaware that they have had one. Because this type of seizure is so subtle and can be over

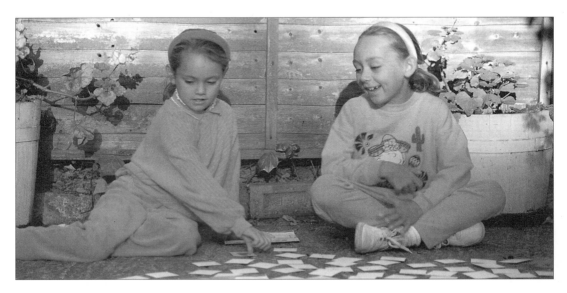

Absences are most commonly seen in childhood or adolescence.

so quickly, it often goes unrecognized, even by the person experiencing it. Some children can have hundreds of these absences every day and, because consciousness is lost during each seizure, their learning can often be quite badly affected. If you can imagine a child being in a basic maths class and the teacher says, 'Two plus two equals four and two plus four equals six,' but the child hears only 'Two plus two [ABSENCE] equals six,' you can see how confusing life could be for that child.

How can I tell if it's an absence?

In order to manage absence seizures, you have to be able to recognize when they are happening. They are most commonly first spotted at school, because there young people are in a situation where they are observed concentrating for longer periods of time than they would be at home. In some instances children may have been having absences unnoticed at home and it is not until they reach school age that it is realized something is not right. Nevertheless, at school it can still be very difficult for a teacher to be able to distinguish between whether a child is having an absence or is simply not paying attention.

If teachers have any suspicions that a particular child may be experiencing absences, there are a number of things they can do. They can keep an eye on the child to see how often these episodes may be happening. They can also discuss their concerns with the child's parents to see if they have noticed anything at home. One simple test is to call the child's name: if the child is simply day-dreaming, he or she will respond to this; but if the child is

having an absence, he or she will be unconscious and will not be able to hear or see anything. This is not foolproof, however, because such a seizure can be over so quickly that it may have stopped just as the end of the child's name was being called, and thus he or she may still be able to respond. It is also important to be aware that, as well as being unable to fulfil their potential at school, children experiencing absences may find it harder mixing with others in their class, possibly showing uncharacteristic signs of shyness. Teachers or parents who are still concerned should discuss the situation with their doctor who may refer the child to a specialist to have further tests carried out (see the section on diagnostic tests, page 17).

How can I help?

Usually no help needs to be given. Occasionally, however, if someone is walking along when they have an absence, they may continue walking even though they are unconscious. Stay with them to make sure that they are not going to hurt themselves and guide them away from any danger.

Myoclonic seizure

The term 'myoclonic' comes from the Greek words *myos*, meaning muscle, and *klonos*, meaning tumult. The arms, head and sometimes the whole body suddenly jerk and the person will lose consciousness for that brief moment. If the person is standing up when the seizure occurs, they may be thrown off balance. Myoclonic seizures often occur in the morning, particularly in the first few hours after waking up.

Types of epileptic seizure

How can I help?

Usually, because these seizures are so short-lived, there is really very little that can be done other than reassure the person when the seizure is over. If the seizure causes the person to be thrown off balance, they may need to be steadied to prevent them falling. If they do fall, check that they haven't hurt themselves.

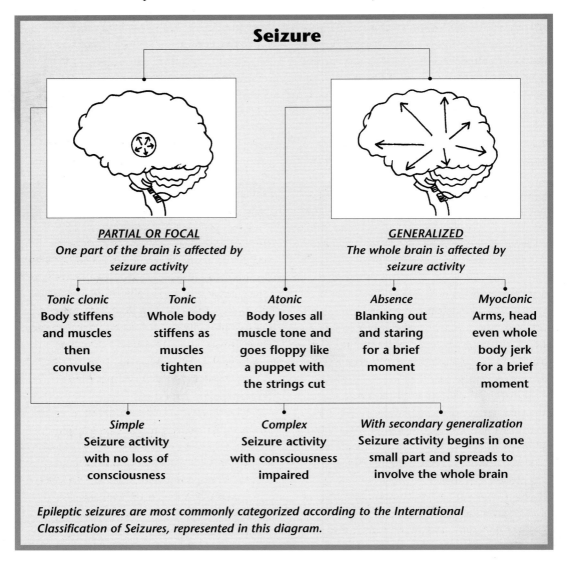

Seizure

PARTIAL OR FOCAL
One part of the brain is affected by seizure activity

GENERALIZED
The whole brain is affected by seizure activity

Tonic clonic
Body stiffens and muscles then convulse

Tonic
Whole body stiffens as muscles tighten

Atonic
Body loses all muscle tone and goes floppy like a puppet with the strings cut

Absence
Blanking out and staring for a brief moment

Myoclonic
Arms, head even whole body jerk for a brief moment

Simple
Seizure activity with no loss of consciousness

Complex
Seizure activity with consciousness impaired

With secondary generalization
Seizure activity begins in one small part and spreads to involve the whole brain

Epileptic seizures are most commonly categorized according to the International Classification of Seizures, represented in this diagram.

Partial or focal seizures

Simple partial seizure

When only a small isolated part of the brain is affected by epileptic activity, a simple partial seizure may occur. When someone experiences this type of seizure, they will be aware of everything that is going on. They may feel a tingling sensation or twitching in an isolated part of the body or have strange feelings in the stomach. They may be able to smell strange smells or have an odd taste in their mouth. What the seizure looks and feels like will depend on which part of the brain is affected. Because a simple partial seizure is so subtle, it is possible that only the person experiencing it will know that it is happening at all. Simple partial seizures sometimes develop into other sorts of seizure and they are then called an 'aura' or referred to as a 'warning'.

Complex partial seizure

Complex partial seizures may take many different forms. During this type of seizure the person will not be totally aware of what they are doing and often act in a very confused way. They may fiddle with their clothing or even undress. Others may behave strangely, rubbing their hands together, lip smacking or chewing. They may wander around a room aimlessly picking up objects and staring at them as if they'd never seen them before. Others may experience strong emotional states or feel that they have no idea where they are despite the fact they are in surroundings normally very familiar to them. They may speak, but what is said doesn't make any sense or they may

vaguely respond to someone speaking to them but in a confused way. Bystanders often don't recognize these actions as being part of an epileptic seizure, particularly if it occurs in a public place, and misunderstandings can result.

How can I help?

Remember that there is nothing you can do to bring the seizure to an end. Simply stay with the person, not restraining them but guiding them away from danger if necessary. Speak calmly and reassuringly and wait with them until they feel they can return to what they were doing before the seizure began.

Status epilepticus

In the great majority of cases an epileptic seizure ends of its own accord, because as soon as the brain 'realizes' what is happening it will stop it. However, on rare occasions a seizure does not stop of its own accord, and this is called status epilepticus. Someone can be said to be 'in status' either when a seizure is prolonged, lasting for a longer period of time than usual, or when one seizure follows

---

Status epilepticus

Status epilepticus is a rare medical condition. However, it is important to be aware that if someone has been into status before, it is more likely that they will do so again.

Types of epileptic seizure

another in quick succession without full recovery in between. Status epilepticus can occur with all the different seizure types. If someone has, say, a partial seizure which makes their left arm jerk, it may simply not stop but may go on for hours. This might be very annoying for the person experiencing the seizure, but it would not be a medical emergency. The individual would probably go to their doctor who would give them medication to make the seizure stop. What must be treated as a medical emergency, however, is if someone has a generalized seizure during which their breathing is impaired, which could result in brain damage if not treated promptly. This is particularly true in children whose immature brains are much more vulnerable than those of adults. In this type of case medical help needs to be called immediately. There is more information on the treatment of status in Chapter four under the heading 'Emergency treatment'.

How do you know if a seizure is going on for too long?

It is not easy to tell whether a seizure has been going on for too long, because what may be a long seizure for one person can be quite normal for someone else. Knowing how long someone's seizure usually lasts will, therefore, help. If the seizure is still going on for two or three minutes after it has usually ended, that is the time to call for medical help. So, for example, if someone whose tonic clonic seizure normally lasts for two minutes is still having that seizure five minutes after it started, call for medical help. If, however, the person always

has seizures of eight minutes, but this time it is going on for ten or eleven minutes, medical assistance should be summoned.

The difficulty arises, of course, when it is not known how long the person's seizures usually last. In such a case help should be summoned if the seizure has not stopped after five or six minutes.

When someone having a seizure comes out of it but goes into another one almost immediately, medical assistance should be summoned, because very often, if this happens, it is more than likely that seizures will start and stop in quick succession for some time. Again, because breathing is not able to return to normal between each seizure, this is a medical emergency and needs to be medically treated.

When to call emergency medical help

Call for medical help immediately if:
- someone has injured themselves badly in a seizure;
- they are having trouble breathing after the seizure;
- the seizure does not stop or another one quickly follows the last.

Either call an ambulance, or if there is someone who is trained to give emergency treatment to the person concerned, alert them to the situation.

Chapter four
How is epilepsy treated?

So it's epilepsy – what now?

Having made a diagnosis of epilepsy and having classified the type or types of seizure, the doctor will usually suggest starting drug treatment. Some young people become anxious when they are told that they are going to be 'put on drugs' for their epilepsy, because they associate the word with illegal drugs; it can therefore be helpful initially to refer to anti-epileptic drugs as anti-epileptic medication. In this chapter drug treatment will be referred to in both ways. Another term sometimes used is anti-convulsant drugs, but this is misleading because anti-epileptic medication controls both convulsive and non-convulsive seizures.

Before prescribing anti-epileptic medication, the doctor will take a number of factors into account:

● Does the person have any other medical condition and if so how is it being treated?
● Has the person ever had any psychiatric problems?
● How often does the person have seizures?
● Are the seizures triggered by alcohol or drug abuse?
● Is the person willing to take medication?

Some doctors prescribe medication immediately while others wait until further tests have been made.

Before going on to look at anti-epileptic drug treatment in more depth, let us consider the answer to another commonly asked question.

Do I have to take anti-epileptic drugs?

Well, of course, the straight answer to this question is no, because no one has to take medication if they do not want to. However, it is vitally important that a decision not to take anti-epileptic medication is made wisely and for all the right reasons. Such a decision can be made only if the person is aware of all the implications – in other words they have been given all the information possible before making their choice. The situation should be discussed with the doctors concerned and talking things over with someone on an epilepsy helpline or with a specialist nurse will also help.

How is epilepsy treated?

Some people may consider not taking anti-epileptic medication if:

● their seizures are few and far between, and when they do occur do not affect their way of life at all;

● they do not drive and don't need to learn to drive;

● having seizures doesn't affect their schooling, career choices or employment;

● they are at little or no risk of badly injuring themselves.

Those who still have seizures, however, are at an increased risk from a phenomenon called sudden unexpected death. It is still not understood why a very small number of people each year die suddenly for no known reason or why people with epilepsy seem more prone to this than others. But it is known that those people who still have seizures are the group most at risk. More information is available from the doctor or from epilepsy organizations.

Some people with epilepsy find their own ways of controlling their seizures without taking medication. This subject is discussed later in this chapter under the heading 'Complementary therapies' (page 50). The fact remains, though, that most people with epilepsy – between 70 and 80 per cent – will achieve total control of their seizures with the right anti-epileptic drug. It is for this reason that most will be recommended by the doctor to start anti-epileptic medication as soon after diagnosis as possible.

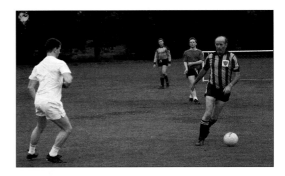

Most people with epilepsy won't actually have seizures because these are controlled by the medication they take.

Drug compliance

The most common reasons for prescribed anti-epileptic medication being ineffective are that it is either not taken at all or not taken in the way it should be. Perhaps the person does not want to displease the doctor, so gets the prescribed drug but fails to take it – perhaps because they are fearful of side effects or don't want to believe they have epilepsy and so don't think they need treatment. Perhaps they have not had an appropriate explanation of why they need the medication and how it works, so they don't understand how and why they need to take it. In some instances someone may simply forget to take their medication at certain times during the day or not remember the instructions they were given accurately enough.

What anti-epileptic medication will the doctor prescribe?

The kind of medication prescribed will depend on the type or types of seizure. This is why it is important for the doctor to have as much detail as possible about the seizures, as a wrong decision about the type or types may mean that the wrong sort of medication is prescribed and seizures will, therefore, not be controlled. If someone has had uncontrolled seizures for many years despite medication, they may be referred for specialist medical assessment. It is possible that correct identification of seizure type and a change in medication may bring good control.

An ever-increasing number of anti-epileptic medications is available, and the table on pages 38–9 gives some brief information about the most commonly used ones. You will see that most drugs have at least two names: an official (chemical or generic) name and a trade (brand) name given by the manufacturer of the drug.

You will also notice that the table is divided into two sections. First-line drugs are those which are used preferably on their own; these are the ones which the doctor will try first. Second-line drugs are those used together with a first-line drug as 'add on' treatment if the first-line drug cannot control the seizures on its own. The doctor will usually try one first-line drug after another if seizures continue, weaning off one and starting the next before using the second-line medication.

The drugs are listed in alphabetical order within each section.

It is important to remember that names and formulations of anti-epileptic drugs may differ from country to country. For example, phenytoin has the brand name Epanutin in the UK but is known as Dilantin in the USA and Australia. Drugs which have licences in some countries may not be licensed in others.

Further information on drugs

If you want more specific information about anti-epileptic drugs, you can talk to your doctor or pharmacist or the information pharmacist at the hospital. Remember: anti-epileptic medication is available on *free* prescription in the UK.

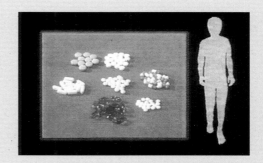

How is epilepsy treated?

FIRST-LINE ANTI-EPILEPTIC DRUGS				
Generic name (brand name in brackets)	**Made by**	**Average daily dose range for adults**	**Use**	**Available as**	**Possible side effects**
Carbamazepine (Tegretol)	Ciba-Geigy	600–1600mg divided into up to 4 doses a day	Effective against generalized tonic clonic and partial seizures. Ineffective against absences. Also used to treat trigeminal neuralgia and some psychiatric conditions	Tablet and suspension form. Slow-release formulation called Tegretol Retard	Double vision, unsteadiness and nausea may occur initially or if the dose is too high. Skin rash is an allergic reaction which affects a small minority of people but necessitates the drug to be stopped
Ethosuximide (Zarontin) (Emeside)	Parke-Davis LAB	1000–1500mg divided into up to 3 doses a day	Effective against absences only	Capsules and syrup	Nausea, drowsiness, headache and stomach upset may occur initially or if the dose is too high. Occasionally may worsen generalized tonic clonic seizures and rarely causes skin rash or depression
Lamotrigine (Lamictal)	Wellcome	200–400mg (or, if also taking sodium valproate, 100–200mg) divided into 2 doses a day	Recommended in partial and generalized tonic clonic seizures where previous treatment has been ineffective	Tablets	Drowsiness, double vision, dizziness and headache. Skin rash is an allergic reaction necessitating stopping the drug
Phenytoin (Epanutin)	Parke-Davis	200–500mg divided into up to 2 doses a day	Effective against generalized tonic clonic and partial seizures. Ineffective against absences	Chewable tablets, capsules and suspension	Drowsiness, unsteadiness and slurred speech may occur if the dose is too high. Very rarely causes allergic skin rashes necessitating the drug to be stopped. Prolonged treatment can be associated with coarsening of facial features, overgrowth of gums or acne
Sodium valproate (Epilim)	Sanofi-Winthrop	500–2000mg divided into up to 2 doses a day	Effective against generalized tonic clonic and partial seizures and absences	Chewable tablets, tablets, sugar-free liquid and syrup. Slow-release formulation called Epilim Chrono	Drowsiness and tremor, irritability and confusion are infrequent side effects. A small number of people may experience hair loss or weight gain which is usually reversible once the dose is reduced. Liver and pancreas damage are rare complications and normally spotted early in treatment

SECOND-LINE ANTI-EPILEPTIC DRUGS

Generic name (brand name in brackets)	Made by	Average daily dose range for adults	Use	Available as	Possible side effects
Clobazam (Frisium)	Hoechst	10–30mg divided into 1 or 2 doses a day	Effective against generalized tonic clonic and partial seizures, but this may wear off over time if used on a day-to-day basis as tolerance develops. Women who have seizures at the time of their periods may be prescribed this medication to take around this time. Also used to treat anxiety	Capsules	Drowsiness and sedation
Clonazapam (Rivotril)	Roche	0.5–3mg divided into 2 doses a day	Effective against partial seizures, absences and myoclonic jerks, but this usually wears off as tolerance develops. Also used to treat anxiety	Tablets	Drowsiness and sedation. A small number of people experience irritability and mental changes and hypersalivation occurs in a few young children
Gabapentin (Neurontin)	Parke-Davis	900–2400mg divided into 3 doses a day	Recommended in partial seizures where previous treatment has been ineffective	Tablets	Drowsiness, dizziness, headaches and fatigue
Phenobarbitone (Gardenal) (Luminal)	May & Baker Sanofi-Winthrop	30–180mg divided into up to 2 doses a day	Effective against generalized tonic clonic and partial seizures	Tablets	Tiredness, sedation and mental slowing may occur even in low doses. In the elderly restlessness and depression is sometimes seen and children may exhibit hyperactivity
Primidone (Mysoline)	ICI	500–1000mg divided into 2 doses a day	Effective against generalized tonic clonic and partial seizures. Not effective against absences and myoclonic jerks	Tablets and suspension	As primidone is partly metabolized as phenobarbitone in the body, side effects are similar to the above. Advisable to start in very low doses as nausea and vomiting may initially occur
Vigabatrin (Sabril)	Marion Merrell Dow	1000–4000mg divided into 2 doses a day	Recommended in partial and secondarily generalized seizures where previous treatment has been ineffective	Tablets and sachets	Drowsiness, nausea, behaviour and mood changes. Psychotic reactions have been reported, so this drug is not usually prescribed for someone with a history of psychiatric problems

How is epilepsy treated?

Emergency treatment

As already stated in Chapter three, status epilepticus is a medical emergency requiring prompt medical intervention especially in children. The drug currently most commonly used for this condition is diazepam (Valium), which is can be injected intravenously by a doctor, or given rectally by a nurse or other trained person (such as a member of the family).

How do anti-epileptic drugs work?

Unlike some other sorts of medication, anti-epileptic drugs control the symptoms of the condition rather than working to cure the cause. They do this by raising the person's

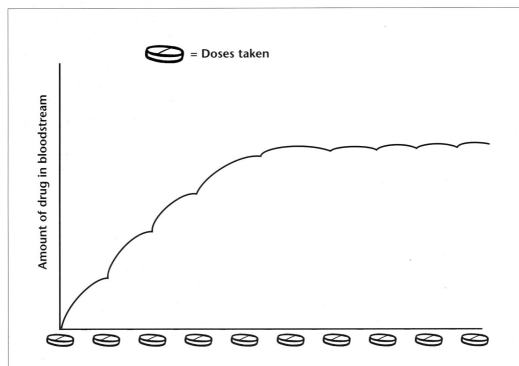

Each time medication is taken the level of the drug in the bloodstream increases until it eaches a level called 'steady state'.

seizure threshold – in other words, by reducing their vulnerability to having seizures. They help increase the brain's 'braking' power or reduce the tendency of the neurones to fire in the excessive way which causes a seizure to occur. To raise the seizure threshold, the drug has to build up to a certain level in the bloodstream and then to be kept at that level by a regular intake. This level is known as steady state. The doctor may first prescribe a low dose and build it up so that the body gets used to the drug gradually, thus lessening the likelihood of side effects. Some people may, however, still experience side effects in the first few days of starting the medication while the body gets used to it, after which time the side effects will disappear.

Once 'steady state' has been reached, the drug should become effective. If, however, it fails to control seizures, the doctor may recommend increasing the dose to see if it is simply that more of the drug is needed. If the person continues to have seizures, the doctor may increase the medication further again until either the seizures are controlled or side effects are experienced. Some people may have an increase in seizures if the dose is too high. At this point the drug will be reduced and another first-line drug will be started at a low level and increased as the other drug is decreasing, providing an overlap of treatment.

Because everyone responds differently to medications and because everyone's epilepsy is individual to them, the doctor usually cannot predict how successful any treatment will be until the person has tried it. There is clearly an element of trial and error in this process, as well as a careful balancing of seizure control on the one hand and the undesirable side effects on the other. Some people are luckier than others in that their seizures are controlled by the first drug they try. Others may have to try many different drugs to get the same control and this could take a year or even longer.

What if I miss a dose?

It is easy to miss a dose of prescribed medication and this often causes great anxiety, especially if someone cannot recall whether they have taken it or not. The thing to remember is that the drug level in the blood needs to be kept as steady as possible and taking the medication reliably as prescribed is, therefore, very important. One missed dose on a rare occasion, however, is unlikely to be dangerous or result in seizures. The exact time of the dose is far less important than the time interval between each one, so if only a short period of time has passed before it is realized that the medication has not been taken, it is usually best to take it. If, however, it is close to the time of the next dose, simply take that next dose, not both doses. One of the best ways to avoid confusion is to keep the medication in a drug wallet. Not only does it help you to remember to take your tablets but it also helps prevent you from taking too many by mistake.

How is epilepsy treated?

Keeping a drug wallet

A drug wallet usually contains seven individual trays – one for each day of the week – with compartments for, say, the morning, afternoon and evening of each day. The medication, in capsule or tablet form, can be transferred once a week into each section from the original container. It is then easy to see if the medication for that day has been taken or not. Drug wallets are available from all good chemists, including the pharmacist at the National Society for Epilepsy, and are not expensive.

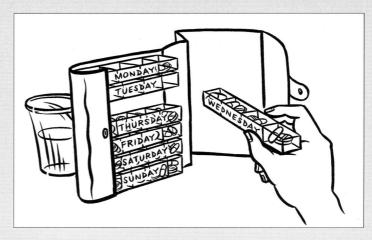

What about side effects?

Any medications we take for any condition have possible side effects and this is also true of anti-epileptic drugs. The doctor cannot tell who will develop either side effects or perhaps an allergic reaction, so it is up to the person taking the anti-epileptic medication to tell the doctor how they feel. It is easier for someone to tell the doctor about side effects if they know what to look out for, and this is especially important for parents of younger children and carers of people with a learning disability who will find it much harder to express how they are feeling.

If either a young child or someone with communication problems is experiencing side effects, their behaviour may change in some way. For example, if someone who cannot communicate is experiencing headaches and double vision, they may become very withdrawn and reluctant to do things or they may become very irritable. Being on the lookout for any change in behaviour at times when drug dosages are being increased or drugs changed will help identify side effects.

If anyone shows an allergic reaction – for

example, a skin rash – it should be reported immediately to the doctor, who may want to stop the drug. It is vitally important not to stop anti-epileptic medication without medical support, however, as stopping abruptly can cause the person to have severe seizures as a reaction and they may go into status (see page 33). Unless someone is allergic to a drug, doctors usually wean them off anti-epileptic drugs slowly over a period of days, weeks or even months.

Most side effects of anti-epileptic drugs are known as 'dose-related' and will disappear once the drug level has been reduced or the drug has been stopped. However, some of the older medications are associated with long-term (chronic) side effects and therefore are not being prescribed as commonly as they once were.

It is necessary for some people to take more than one type of anti-epileptic medication. These people may be more prone to side effects, as are those whose epilepsy has resulted from head injury or brain damage. It is, therefore, even more important to achieve a careful balance between side effects and seizure control. It is in these cases, as well as with certain types of anti-epileptic

Therapeutic drug level monitoring is carried out to discover how much of an anti-epileptic drug is in the bloodstream.

medication in combination, that drug level monitoring is important.

Therapeutic drug level monitoring

Therapeutic drug level monitoring tells the doctor how much of a drug is in the bloodstream. People frequently ask, 'How often should I have a blood test?'. Generally there is no need for drug levels to be tested routinely. However, there are certain circumstances when it is advisable:

● if someone has started experiencing side effects or an increase in seizures;

● if an extra drug is being added or an existing drug is being stopped;

● if a woman taking anti-epileptic medication is pregnant;

● to check that the person is taking the drug as prescribed;

● to check for drug interactions.

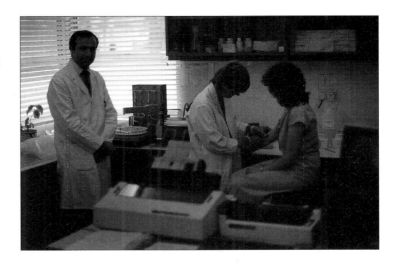

How is epilepsy treated?

Can I take other medications with my anti-epileptic drugs?

Some other prescription medication can either interfere with or be interfered with by anti-epileptic drugs, so it is important to ask your doctor or pharmacist whether the particular drug combination about to be started is suitable. Most other medications can be taken quite safely with anti-epileptic drugs but it is wise to have this confirmed. The same is true of over-the-counter remedies. People who have another medical condition which means that they have to take medication over a long period of time – for example, a heart condition, high or low blood pressure or arthritis – need to be particularly aware that these drugs may potentially interact with the medication they take for their epilepsy. This is especially true for elderly people who may be taking a number of different medications simultaneously. It can be confusing, but it is important to take all medication as prescribed. The doctor and/or pharmacist should be consulted when any form of medical treatment is started for the first time.

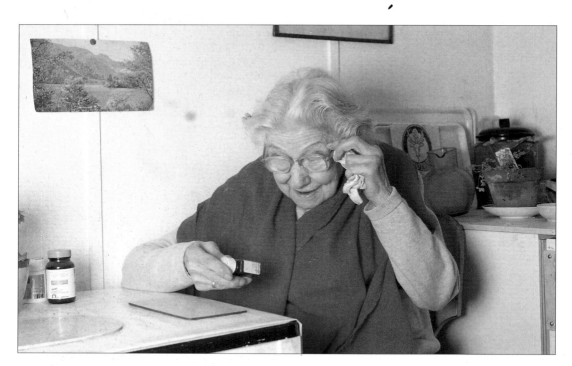

Taking many different forms of medication at any one time can be confusing, but it is very important to take all medication as prescribed.

Contraception

Anti-epileptic medication can make some other drugs less effective and the most notable example of this is the contraceptive pill. A standard 30 microgram oestrogen pill may be inadequate for some women taking anti-epileptic medication. The dose may have to be increased to 50 micrograms a day to offer the same protection.

Is anti-epileptic medication safe during pregnancy?

Many women with epilepsy are concerned about taking anti-epileptic medication during pregnancy and because of this it is important to discuss the issues of starting a family with the doctor well before conception. The doctor can then assess current drug treatment and ensure that the dose is the minimum necessary to control seizures. It is often recommended that all women planning a pregnancy take a folic acid supplement to their diet to reduce the risk of some developmental defects. If any reductions to the anti-epileptic medication are necessary, they should be made well before the pregnancy is planned. It may well be, of course, that the anti-epileptic medication the woman is taking is already at an acceptable dose. All drugs are potentially harmful to the developing foetus and no anti-epileptic drug is entirely safe in pregnancy, but these risks are minimized if the drug treatment is simple. Equally the mother and child are at risk from the mother having

If you are planning to start a family and are taking anti-epileptic medication, discuss this with your doctor well before conception.

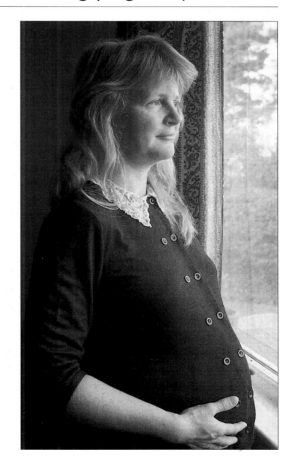

How is epilepsy treated?

seizures during pregnancy. Concerns should be discussed with the doctor, but it must be stressed that the majority of women with epilepsy who take anti-epileptic medication have normal healthy babies. The child will have been exposed to any drugs the mother is taking while in the womb, so there is no reason why the mother should not breast feed the baby if she wants to. If an unplanned pregnancy occurs, it is important to see the doctor as soon as possible: no changes in medication should be made without discussion with the doctor.

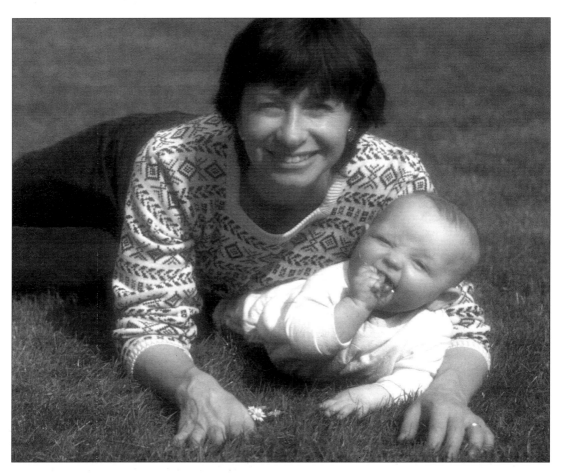

The great majority of women with epilepsy who are taking anti-epileptic medication have perfectly normal healthy babies.

Can I drink alcohol when taking anti-epileptic medication?

Traditionally people with epilepsy have been told to avoid alcohol altogether, but unless either the doctor has given a particular reason why alcohol should not be drunk or the person with epilepsy knows that even the smallest amount of alcohol causes them a problem, there is no reason why alcohol cannot be enjoyed in moderation. Some people with epilepsy find that drinking even small amounts of alcohol can cause them to have more seizures than they would normally, but most people can drink socially without experiencing any problems with their seizures at all.

What is a moderate intake of alcohol?

3 units per day for a man
2 units per day for a woman

1 unit equals:
- ¹/2 pint beer or lager
- 1 glass of white wine
- 1 single measure of spirits
- 1 small glass of sherry

What about stopping drug treatment?

If someone hasn't had any seizures for two or more years, their doctor may suggest that they slowly come off the medication to find out if they actually need to take it any longer, as it is possible that the epilepsy has simply gone away. There is no way of testing for this other than coming off medication, but before doing so the person needs to think very carefully about how their life would be affected if, once off medication, they started to have seizures again (particularly if they are reliant on a driving licence – see Chapter six). Although the doctor may have suggested stopping drug treatment, it is totally up to the individual whether they decide to do this or not. Many people with epilepsy decide to stay on medication for many years simply because they do not want to risk having further seizures.

If someone does take the doctor's advice and come off medication, it must be done very slowly, reducing the dose over a long period of time and with full medical support. If seizures do recur, the person will need to go back on their anti-epileptic medication. However, there is a slight risk in this case that the same medication that was taken before may not control the seizures as it once did, although the reasons for this are unknown.

Remember:

Coming off medication too quickly and without medical support can be very dangerous, causing severe seizures and sometimes status epilepticus (see page 33).

How is epilepsy treated?

Alternatives to drug treatment

Epilepsy surgery: what is it and who can be helped by it?

To put it very simply, epilepsy surgery involves the removal of the part of the brain which is causing the epilepsy, and it still remains the only cure for the condition. It is clear, therefore, that the people who are considered for this form of treatment have to be shown to be suitable. To establish this the person will need to be referred to a specialist. There are a number of criteria which the doctors concerned will take into account when assessing someone's suitability for surgery. Some of these criteria are listed below, though not necessarily in order of priority.

● All drug treatment has been tried and has been found to be unsuccessful or unsuitable.

● There is evidence to show that seizures are arising from one localized area of the brain.

● The person's life would be dramatically improved by becoming seizure-free or having a reduction in seizure frequency.

● The part of the brain that would need to be removed is accessible – that is, that no other areas of the brain would be damaged in the process of removing it.

● The person would be able to function totally normally without this section of the brain.

● It is highly unlikely that the areas of the brain responsible for sight, hearing, movement or speech would be damaged during the operation. If the area is close to these parts of the brain, the risk would probably be considered too great.

● The person must, of course, be healthy and not have any other medical problems which would make them unsuitable for this type of major surgery.

To establish some of the above there is a number of tests which may need to be carried out, including MRI and PET scans and video telemetry as well as psychological tests. It may well be that the doctors cannot say how suitable someone is for surgery until at least some of the tests have been carried out. Someone who has been told that surgery is an option for them is bound to want more information about what is involved. Contacting an epilepsy helpline, discussing the situation with a specialist nurse or other people who have had the surgery will help them to put together the questions they need to ask their specialist. It's advisable to write down the questions so that they are not forgotten. They may include:

● What exactly does the operation involve?

● How long will the operation take?

● How long will I need to recuperate?

● How soon afterwards will I be able to work?

● How likely is it that I will be seizure-free after the operation?

● Will I still need to take medication and if so for how long?

● What sort of risks are involved?

Noting down the answers to the questions is also a good idea as then they can be referred to at a later date. Having been given this information, it is up to the person concerned to decide if they want to proceed with the operation.

Although only a small number of people with epilepsy will be suitable for epilepsy surgery, it is highly successful for the majority who undergo this form of treatment: a high percentage become seizure-free.

Vagus nerve stimulation (VNS)

As yet only a small number of people with epilepsy have been treated by VNS and of these just a small percentage have had a significant reduction in the number of seizures experienced. Only as more people try this alternative form of treatment will it be known how successful it is. VNS, as the name implies, is a mild electrical stimulation of a nerve called the vagus nerve which carries information to and from the brain and which is thought to be connected to the parts of the brain which may be involved when a seizure occurs. A special lead is attached to the vagus nerve at one end

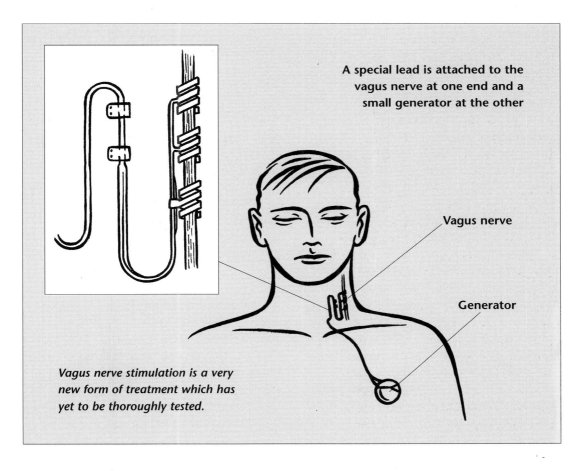

A special lead is attached to the vagus nerve at one end and a small generator at the other

Vagus nerve

Generator

Vagus nerve stimulation is a very new form of treatment which has yet to be thoroughly tested.

How is epilepsy treated?

and to a small generator at the other. This generator sends bursts of electrical stimulation to the vagus nerve. It is thought that VNS works by stimulating the nerve which disrupts the pathways used during a seizure. More research is needed to discover how helpful this method of treatment actually is for people with epilepsy generally.

Complementary therapies and alternative medicine: are these helpful for people with epilepsy?

The most successful treatment for the control of seizures is anti-epileptic drug treatment achieving total control of seizures in between 70 and 80 per cent of people with epilepsy. And it is in the area of drug treatment that most research is carried out. Research into other complementary and alternative therapies and techniques which may help people with epilepsy, although far less well supported and funded, is also going on, but its findings are often inconclusive because only a small number of people have taken part or the results are 'anecdotal', based on what people have said they have found rather than being proven. There is growing interest in this area, however, and it will be interesting to see what research reveals in the future and how these complementary and alternative therapies and techniques will be able to help people with epilepsy.

The addresses of some organizations concerned with complementary and alternative therapies (although the National Society for Epilepsy is unable to endorse them) are listed on page 79.

What sort of other therapies or treatments are there?

The forms of therapies and treatments outlined below are the ones which people most commonly ask about. But when considering any form of therapy it is crucial to make sure that the person advising on the treatment is appropriately qualified. Contacting the head office of the particular association or body concerned with the treatment and asking them to recommend someone locally will help to ensure this.

It is also vitally important that any such treatment does not interfere with the prescribed anti-epileptic medication. The doctor who prescribed the anti-epileptic medication should be consulted and the practitioner who will be starting the complementary therapy should be told exactly what their patient is taking for their epilepsy. Again, it must be stressed that if someone is considering coming off their anti-epileptic medication they *must* do so with their doctor's support. Stopping anti-epileptic medication too quickly or in the wrong way can be dangerous and may result in the person going into status epilepticus (see page 33).

Yoga and meditation

Yoga and meditation are good techniques to learn and practise to help prevent the occurrence of seizures which may be brought on by stress. About 30 per cent of people with epilepsy find they have an increased number of seizures when they are under stress and clearly if they can reduce the stress in their lives the number of seizures they experience will lessen.

Aromatherapy

Aromatherapy can also aid relaxation and so reduce the stress which can precipitate seizures. The use of massage generally is recognized as helpful in stress reduction but aromatherapy also uses essential oils which can affect the nervous system. Essential oils, which are taken from plants, concentrated and used in pure form, are diluted with a 'carrier' oil and massaged into the skin. Different oils have different properties and thus can achieve different effects.

It is known that some oils have epileptogenic qualities; that is, that they can cause seizures in someone who is susceptible. It is also recognized that some may have the opposite effect.

Oils people with epilepsy should avoid

Hyssop ● Rosemary
Sweet fennel ● Sage

It is important to be treated by an appropriately qualified aromatherapist as only they will know which oils should not be used for people with epilepsy.

Oils which may be helpful

Ylang ylang ● Camomile ● Lavender

Biofeedback

Biofeedback is based on the theory that someone knows when they are about to have a seizure because they have aura or warning (that is, a simple partial seizure), which then develops into another type of seizure (either complex partial or tonic clonic). Some people can learn a technique which may delay the following seizure or even prevent it from happening at all. They may learn to do this over time without needing to be taught how to do it. For example, someone whose simple partial seizures take the form of a tingling in the arm may find that rubbing that arm can sometimes stop their seizure developing into a tonic clonic type.

It is being suggested, however, that some people can be taught how to recognize the start of their seizure or warning and the therapist and the individual can then go on to explore techniques to prevent the seizure spreading. The action someone needs to take to prevent this spread will depend entirely on the sort of simple partial seizure they have as their warning, and so is very individual to that person. Someone can explore this on their own to find out if any particular technique can be of help to them. It should be emphasized that many people with epilepsy will not be able to improve control of their seizures in this way. However, as is discussed in the following chapter, becoming familiar with how epilepsy can affect someone specifically will help in a number of ways.

Chapter five

How can you help yourself?

For most people with epilepsy, seizures happen totally out of the blue with no warning at all. However, others may begin to notice that their seizures are triggered by something quite specific or tend to happen at certain times, and so they can take action to try to lessen the likelihood of them occurring. It is known that some people will be able to recognize a regular pattern in the occurrence of their seizures. Some, for example, have seizures only while they are asleep (which is known as nocturnal epilepsy); others always experience seizures in the first few hours after waking up, or only in the afternoon; others may find that their seizures happen regularly at the end of the week or at certain times of the month.

Getting to know your epilepsy

Clearly, if someone can predict what can cause them to have seizures, or at what times they are most likely to occur, this will be of great help when they are deciding what to do on a day-to-day basis, but also, and most importantly, how having epilepsy may influence their choice of work and their lifestyle generally. So finding out if there is anything predictable about their epilepsy, or whether there are any specific triggers to their seizures, can give someone back the control that having the condition might have taken away.

Nocturnal seizures

The term 'nocturnal seizures' is slightly misleading because it actually refers to seizures which occur only when the person is asleep. They may be asleep at lunchtime and have a seizure then, and this would still be referred to as a nocturnal seizure. If someone is awake at night and has a seizure while they are awake, regardless of how late it is this is *not* a nocturnal seizure because the person is awake when it happens.

It is known that, while we are asleep, the brain works in a certain way which causes some people to have seizures then and then only. If someone knows that they do not have seizures

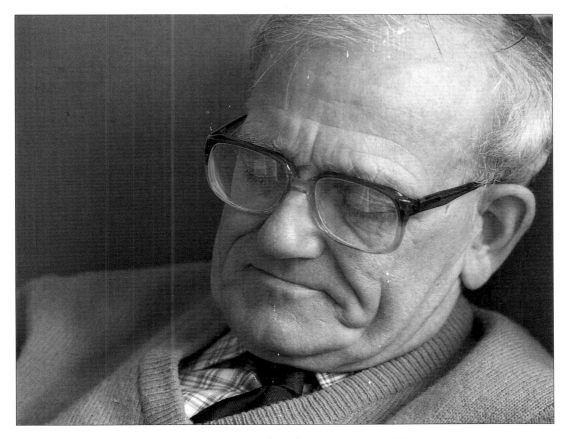

Nocturnal seizures are those which happen during sleep – not just at night.

while they are awake, this will help them a great deal when, for instance, they are applying for jobs and getting a driving licence. There is further discussion on employment and driving in the next chapter.

What can help?

Some people may find that they have more nocturnal seizures when they are overtired or have disturbed their normal sleep patterns by doing shift work or while they have suffered insomnia as a result of a jet lag, for example. Establishing a good sleep routine can, therefore, be helpful in reducing the likelihood of seizures being triggered. Making up for lost sleep as soon as possible, rather than waiting until the following night, will help prevent overtiredness.

How can you help yourself?

Stress

Everyone has stress in their lives and this is not always a bad thing. Even going on holiday can be stressful, at least until you get there, and in fact being excited is technically seen as a sort of 'stress'. But what most people refer to as stress is the 'negative' kind – the sort experienced when going through a difficult time at work or losing a job, when someone close to them dies or when a relationship breaks up. Everyone is likely to face events such as these in their lifetime and they are never easy. But there are other sorts of negative stress which people with epilepsy face because of their condition. Some people decide not to tell anyone that they have epilepsy and live in constant fear that they may be found out. Living with this level of anxiety on a day-to-day basis could make the chance of having a seizure all the more likely. There will, of course, be decisions to be made about whom to tell and whom not to and this can in fact be one of the hardest issues to deal with.

Not knowing very much about epilepsy will also cause stress to someone with the condition when someone else asks them about it. This other individual may be a potential employer at an interview, a friend, relative or prospective partner. It is known from research that many people know little about their epilepsy and know even less about the condition generally, and so find it difficult and embarrassing talking to other people about it. A small number of people with epilepsy find that they have their seizures when they relax – at the end of a working day, at weekends or on holiday. There is no easy solution to this as obviously it is not possible and certainly not advisable not to unwind or take a break! But it can be helpful to know when seizures may occur so that allowances can be made if necessary.

What can help?

Learning a form of recognized relaxation technique, such as yoga or meditation which is done daily, can be very helpful in reducing the effects of stress. As always, it is important to learn from an appropriately qualified person.

Being able to relax is not something which everyone finds easy, but everyone should be able to learn ways in which they can become more relaxed. Identifying what situations are stressful and why will help a person with epilepsy to adopt coping strategies to reduce the likelihood of seizures being triggered. There are also ways of managing stressful situations. For example, when someone feels that they are becoming anxious, they could relax their shoulders and body posture and concentrate on pleasant thought. Someone might want to think of themselves on a beautiful beach with palm trees and a calm blue ocean, and a warm sun in the sky. Others may find that the pleasant thought of walking through a leafy wood filled with bluebells on a warm afternoon with the sun filtering through the trees is a good one to calm them.

There are also various breathing techniques that can be learned to help relieve tension. The family doctor should be able to give advice on both relaxation techniques and stress management.

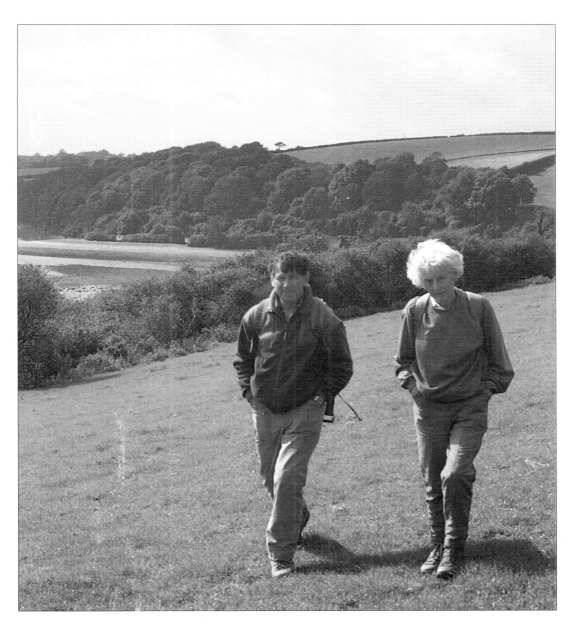

Learning to relax can play an important part in controlling seizures.

How can you help yourself?

Boredom

Being bored is another form of stress and some people are aware that this is the time when they are likely to have seizures. It is recognized that many people, when they are mentally active and enjoying what they are doing, are far less likely to have seizures than if they are not involved in any activity which interests them. This fact is often used by disability employment advisors (who help people with epilepsy and those with other disabilities to find work) when talking to an employer who is concerned about seizures occurring in the work place.

What can help?

People who find boredom a trigger to seizures will clearly find it helpful to take up some pursuit or hobby that is of interest to them. Those who may be particularly affected by boredom, such as children during school holidays, people in some form of residential care and less active elderly people, may need help in getting motivated and choosing what sort of activity to take up. Because having epilepsy can be very isolating, some people with the condition may not have many friends or may find it hard to mix with people. Joining a club or group with common interests or common concerns, or helping a local charity may well provide an answer to the problem of boredom.

Tiredness

It is not uncommon for people with epilepsy to recognize that when they are tired, having not slept well or having missed some sleep, they are more likely to have seizures. As mentioned earlier, shift work and jet lag can cause disturbed sleep patterns and so potentially could cause seizures. Parents particularly may be concerned about their teenage child with epilepsy staying out late and missing sleep if they have to go school, college or work the next morning.

What can help?

Avoiding overtiredness is clearly going to help those whose seizures are likely to be triggered by it, but it is important to make sure that unnecessary restrictions are neither imposed on the person concerned nor self-imposed. Restrictions on someone's lifestyle may do more harm than good if it prevents them living a normal active life. Therefore it is important to assess how overtired someone needs to be before seizures are likely to happen and to look at how restrictive bans on late nights with friends or long flights to exotic locations may actually be to the individual in question. Some people find that as long as they don't stay out late more than two nights in a row, or as long as they sleep when they arrive at a holiday destination rather than staying awake until night-time, some sleep loss or disturbance doesn't actually affect them. It is not uncommon, however, for people affected in this way to avoid doing shift work in an attempt to keep seizures to a minimum, although, of course, this may not always be possible.

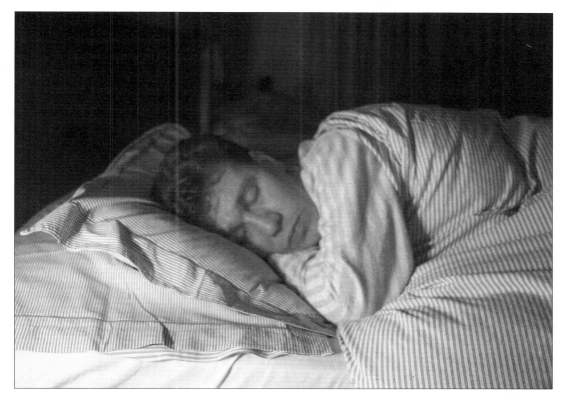

Establishing a regular sleep pattern will prevent overtiredness, which may trigger seizures.

Alcohol

Some people with epilepsy choose to drink no alcohol at all. However, for the majority, social drinking is perfectly acceptable. There is an interaction between alcohol and anti-epileptic medication, but this should not cause a problem if alcohol is taken in moderation. The time when seizures are most likely to happen after drinking is during the 'hangover' phase, usually the following morning, as this is when the seizure threshold is particularly low.

57

How can you help yourself?

Alcohol is the *only* trigger which has this delayed effect; other triggers or 'precipitants' to seizures have an immediate effect. Only with alcohol does the resistance to seizures become low hours afterwards rather than at the time when the person was drinking. Seizures which are triggered by television, for example, happen while the person is actually watching it and not hours later (see 'Photosensitive epilepsy' on page 61).

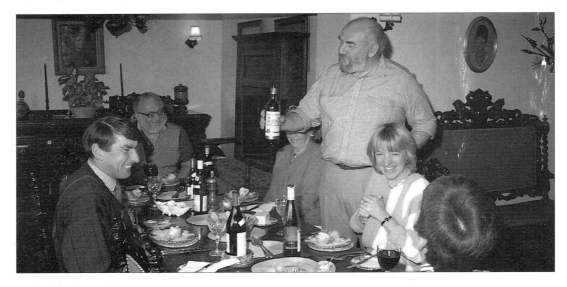

Social drinking can help you relax, but don't overdo it.

Diet

Generally speaking, there has been no evidence at all to show that what someone eats has a direct effect on the number of seizures they have, with two exceptions.

● **The ketogenic diet** is sometimes useful in children with Lennox-Gastaut syndrome and generalized myoclonic seizures. It is very high in fat and oils and tends to be rather unpalatable and not particularly healthy. It can be used for only short periods at a time and tends to have only short-term success. It must be carried out only under medical supervision.

● **Allergy** It is recognized that some people may have an allergy to something they eat which can cause them to have seizures. This is very rare, however, and the person will usually also show other signs of suffering from an allergy.

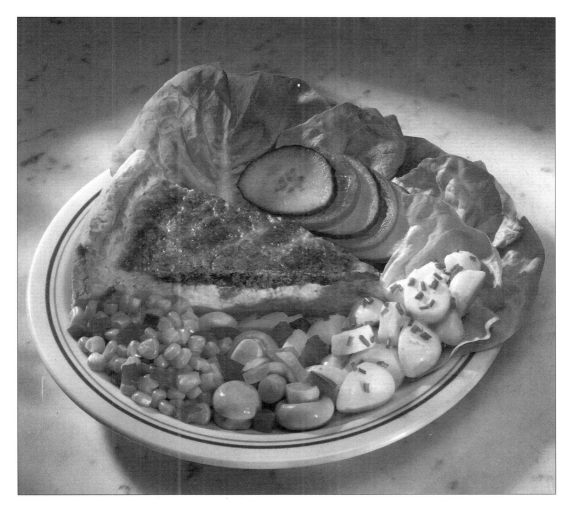

A nutritious well-balanced diet is important for general good health.

If there is no recognized diet for people with epilepsy, what can help?

Eating a good, healthy, balanced diet that includes plenty of fresh vegetables and fruit is beneficial to everyone, including people with epilepsy. Most important is making sure that meals are eaten regularly. Ensuring that no meals are missed may be of more benefit than concentrating on exactly what is eaten.

59

How can you help yourself?

Hormones

It is recognized that some people develop epilepsy or find that their epilepsy goes away at times of their lives when their bodies are undergoing great hormonal changes. Examples of this would be at puberty, during pregnancy and during the menopause. Some women also find that their seizures occur regularly just before or during menstruation, or that the number of seizures will increase at this time.

What can help?

Simply being aware that these hormonal changes can influence someone's epilepsy is important. Women who experience an increase in their number of seizures around the time of menstruation should speak to their doctor, as sometimes taking extra anti-epileptic medication in the week before the menstrual period may be helpful.

Anger

Some people have seizures if they become very angry or frustrated. On rare occasions young children and people with a learning disability have been known to get angry on purpose to bring on a seizure if they want their own way.

What can help?

As with people who find stressful situations a problem, managing the feelings and preventing them from building up to an explosive level will help. Learning to vent frustration and displeasure in an appropriate way at the time when they are initially felt will help prevent feelings of anger being bottled up and so make a seizure less likely to occur. When it is suspected that a seizure has been deliberately brought on, making minimal fuss will lessen the likelihood of it happening again.

Prodrome

Prodrome is a phenomenon which, until quite recently, many doctors did not believe existed because there was no physical proof of its existence. Prodrome is the period of time before a seizure occurs when some people with epilepsy are 'not themselves'. They may be rather irritable for hours, days or, less commonly, weeks before having a seizure. This change in their behaviour may be so subtle that it goes unnoticed by the individual in question and it may be friends or family who spot it.

What can help?

No one can do anything for someone feeling like this other than being understanding, in the same way that they would be if a friend or member of the family had had a disturbed night and were feeling grumpy as a result.

Photosensitive epilepsy

In some people seizures may be triggered by flashing or flickering light, or even by certain geometric shapes and patterns, such as stripes and checks. This is a fairly rare condition and is known as photosensitive epilepsy. Of the one in 200 people who have epilepsy only very few (less than 5 per cent) are photosensitive: the condition is most common in children and adolescents and becomes far less frequent with age, being very uncommon from the mid-20s onwards. Most people with photosensitive epilepsy will have seizures both with and without this trigger and it is quite rare only to have seizures triggered by flashing or flickering lights and at no other time. Photosensitive epilepsy usually responds well to treatment by standard anti-epileptic medication, commonly Epilim (sodium valproate).

How is photosensitive epilepsy diagnosed?

Very often it is the person experiencing the seizures, or members of their family, who will notice that seizures are being triggered by flashing or flickering lights or by particular geometric shapes or patterns. One of the common tests used to diagnose epilepsy is the electroencephalogram (EEG) and part of the standard test is a period of photic stimulation, during which a light is flashed into the person's eyes for a short period of time and at different flash frequencies. If there is any abnormal change in the brainwaves, this will be recorded on the EEG and photosensitive epilepsy may be diagnosed.

What frequency of flashing/flickering light will trigger a seizure?

The frequency of flashing/flickering light most likely to trigger seizures varies from person to person, but the most common is between 5 and 30 flashes per second. Some people will be sensitive to higher flash frequencies and only a very few will be sensitive to a slow flash frequency – that is, below 5 flashes per second.

What are the most common triggers for someone with photosensitive epilepsy?

● Watching television, particularly if it is faulty thereby causing a slow flicker, or if it is not tuned in properly.
● Playing video games or using other computer graphics.
● Sunlight coming through a line of trees.
● Looking out of a window in a fast-moving train.
● Sunlight flickering on water.
● Stroboscopic lights.

Visual display units (VDUs)

VDUs generally operate at a very high flash frequency, so they do not tend to provoke

How can you help yourself?

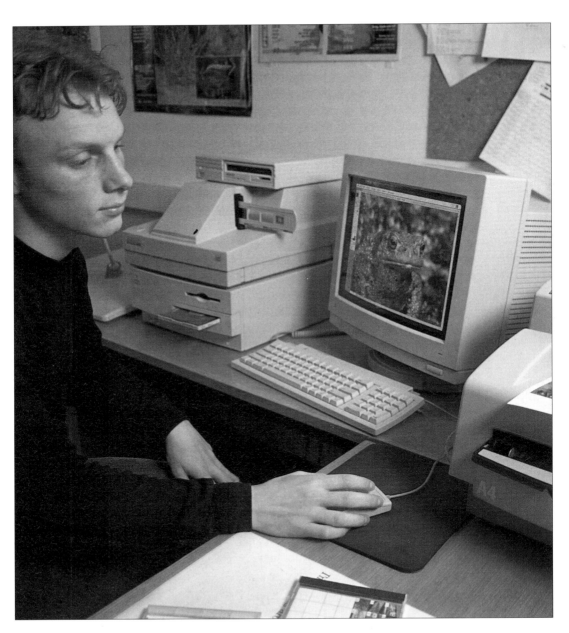

Even in people with photosensitive epilepsy VDUs rarely cause a problem.

seizures in the majority of people with photosensitive epilepsy. However, there are a few people whose seizures are triggered by high flash frequencies and if medication is not controlling the photosensitive epilepsy this could be problematic. What is most important is what is showing on the screen: for example, if there is a flickering or flashing image or a changing geometric pattern, it could be this which is triggering the seizure rather than the flash frequency of the VDU itself.

Computer games

Playing a computer game rarely causes seizures in someone without a known history of epilepsy. Occasionally someone may have their first epileptic seizure while playing a computer game, but usually such an individual would have a tendency to seizures provoked by flashing light – that is, they are photosensitive – which until then had been unrecognized.

Strobe lighting

Many parents are concerned about letting their child go to discos because of the flashing lights used. Stroboscopes certainly can trigger seizures in someone with photosensitive epilepsy, particularly if the background illumination is low, so it may be advisable to avoid this kind of lighting. Local authorities in the UK have guidelines concerning the flash frequency of strobe lighting and the local environmental health department will be able to provide you with further information about this. If a stroboscope is used unexpectedly – as part of a show, for example – covering one eye will reduce the photosensitive effect.

Helpful hints for people with known photosensitivity

● Be aware that tiredness may increase the risk of photosensitive seizures.
● Change channels on the television using a remote control to avoid going too close to the screen. (There is a greater risk of having an epileptic seizure when your field of vision is dominated by the screen.)
● Try to avoid watching faulty televisions or those which are not tuned in properly.
● Consider using a high-frequency (100 hertz) television or one with a small screen.
● Do not sit too close to the television or the VDU.
● Turn down the brightness on a VDU and consider using an anti-glare screen.
● Wear sunglasses to reduce glare.
● If playing a video game, sit as far away from the screen as possible. Do not play when tired or for longer than 20 minutes at a time, and make sure that the background lighting is good.
● It is rare for seizures to be triggered by hand-held miniature screens or by film in a cinema.

Chapter six

Living with epilepsy

How 'having epilepsy' will affect someone's general lifestyle will vary according to the individual and will to a certain extent depend on how successful the medical treatment is in controlling their seizures. However, even if someone no longer has seizures, they will still find that, because they have epilepsy or a history of it, there may be implications in areas of their life such as employment, for example. In this chapter we will look at some of the common day-to-day issues faced by people with epilepsy.

Going to school

Once a child with epilepsy reaches school age, good communication with the teachers at the school is essential. Staff must know how to deal calmly and confidently with any seizures which may happen during school hours. The teachers may not know very much about epilepsy, so discussing it with them will help them to understand what the child is going through and why. It will also make it easier for them to explain about epilepsy to the other children in the class. Telling other children can be a very sensitive subject for the child with epilepsy, so the whole issue of whom to tell and how needs to be discussed and agreed beforehand.

Some children with epilepsy may feel isolated because they feel they are different. Every effort should be made to treat them in the same way as other children: they should be exposed to the same chances of success and failure in both academic and physical subjects. It is important that parents and teachers alike do not have unrealistically low or high expectations of the child's ability and also ensure that they are given the same rewards and punishments as other children. If this is not the case, the child may be seen as different by the other children and become frustrated at not being able to do what the others are doing. The child may equally feel that he or she can get away with more, but it should be remembered that the side effects of medication can include hyperactivity, which will obviously affect the way the child behaves. If this is suspected, the doctor should be consulted rather than the child blamed for his or her behaviour. Teachers also need to be aware that subtle seizures may occur and to watch out for them. If they do notice anything, they should

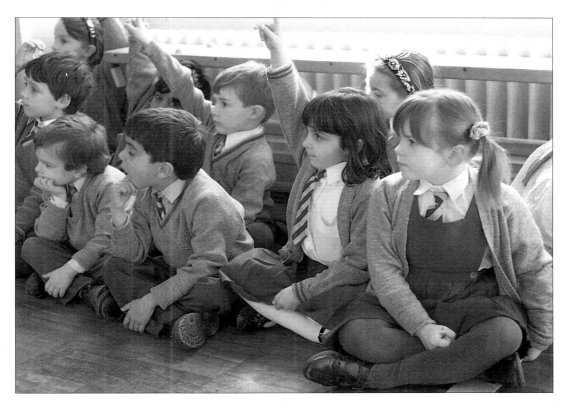

Every effort should be made to treat children with epilepsy in the same way as other children.

pass this information to the parents so that the doctor can be informed.

In the UK, if a child has had changes in medication and evaluation by a specialist but still shows signs of problems with school work or behaviour, his or her needs can be 'statemented'. Parents or teachers can start this process, which will involve the gathering of much information from the doctor, parents and teachers and may also involve a psychologist who will give a series of tests to find out in which areas the child is experiencing problems and why. The written document finally produced is called the statement. Recommendations will be made in the statement about the child's needs and how these can be met at school. The local education authority is then legally bound to make any appropriate educational provision for the child which is necessary.

Appropriate career advice should be given well before the young person leaves school either for full-time employment or to go on to higher education.

Living with epilepsy

Going to work

How or if someone's employment or employment prospects will be affected by their having epilepsy will depend on two main factors:
● the nature of the epilepsy – the type of seizures and how often they occur;
● the nature of the employment – the type of work the person is doing or wants to do.

Having epilepsy does not stop people from working, but it may influence the type of work they do or the way they go about finding employment. In the UK there are only a very few occupations which are closed to people with epilepsy and these include:
● being an airline pilot;
● joining the Royal Navy;
● working in the fire service in an active capacity;
● being a train driver;
● working on track maintenance for London Underground.

There are certain jobs which, although not closed to people with a history of epilepsy, do have restrictions on them. For example, in the UK, to be a professional driver and to hold a large goods vehicle (LGV) or passenger carrying vehicle (PCV) licence, someone has to have been totally free of seizures *and* not taking anti-epileptic medication for at least ten years. (In the USA this period can vary from three months to one year, according to the state legislature, although in some states there is no set seizure-free period and everyone is judged individually on their doctor's recommendation.) For more information on driving see page 69. Jobs in the police force, working with young children or teaching posts which involve physical education, cookery or science subjects all have restrictions, as do midwifery and intensive-care nursing jobs.

However, the longer someone has been seizure-free, the more training and employment prospects are open to them. Once someone has had seizure control for one to two years, nurse or teacher training becomes possible. Once seizure-free (while awake) for a year, they can hold a driving licence and more jobs become a possibility, and of course getting to work can become easier.

How do I go about getting a job?

As for anyone job hunting, the most useful approach is to look through advertisements in newspapers and magazines and go to the Job Centre. Choosing employment to suit your level of qualifications, skills and abilities is vitally important and success in selecting the right sort of jobs to apply for will clearly determine success in getting a job. Of course, if someone has epilepsy, it needs to be taken into account, but if there are no statutory barriers or specific restrictions in place for people with a history of epilepsy, and particularly if someone has been seizure-free for a year or more, 'having epilepsy' should not be an issue.

If someone is still having seizures, however, the kind of work they can apply for will depend on the type and frequency of their seizures as well as any risks having one in the workplace might present to them and their colleagues. As this varies so much from person to person and from job to job, specific queries or concerns need to be talked over individually. The person's doctor may be able to give advice on this and epilepsy helplines can also be a valuable source of help. If you live in the UK the Employment Medical Advisory Service (EMAS), which is available to individuals as well as employers and occupational health personnel, will give a free and confidential opinion about particular types of work where epilepsy is involved. The disability employment advisor (DEA) at the Job Centre, whose task it is to help people with disabilities to find work, can access a number of different services. How much particular DEAs know about epilepsy will depend on their training and experience, but the epilepsy organizations are happy to provide DEAs with any information they may need when helping a client with epilepsy.

Filling in the application form

When applying for a job, some people question writing 'epilepsy' in the section of the form requesting medical history as they fear their application could be rejected simply because of this. There are various options to consider and the individual should decide which one they feel most happy with. One option is to leave this part of the form blank and to discuss the epilepsy during the interview. Another alternative is simply to state nothing about the epilepsy but to write 'to be discussed at interview'. Finally this part of the form can be completed with brief and positive information about the epilepsy. For example:

 Do you have or have you ever had any long-term illness, disease or medical condition?

 I used to have seizures but the medication I have taken for the last year and a half has controlled them completely and so this will not affect my ability to do this job in any way. (Some doctors are happy to write a letter outlining their patient's current medical situation and if this is helpful it can be attached to the application form, or it can be suggested to the potential employer that further medical information can be obtained from the doctor. Check well beforehand that your doctor is willing to supply this.)

Attending the interview

If someone has been called to a job interview and has not declared their epilepsy on the application form, this is an opportunity to inform the interviewer of the fact that they have epilepsy. It can be done towards the end of the interview once the person has 'sold' themselves and their skills and abilities. Even if the employer already knows that the interviewee has epilepsy, he or she may still want to ask questions about it. It is therefore very important that the interviewee is able to give a brief, to-the-point and positive impression of their condition. It may need practice to do this, so role-playing an interview situation with someone beforehand may help. Having some basic knowledge about epilepsy in general can also be useful.

Living with epilepsy

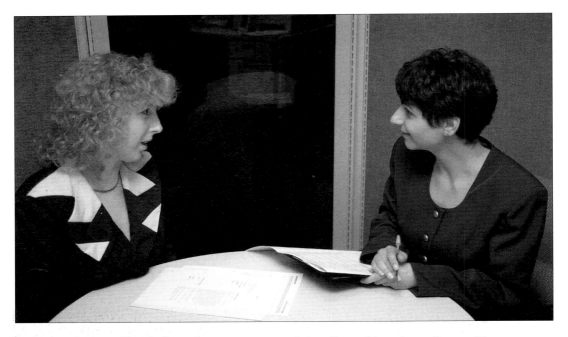

The job interview offers the interviewee an opportunity to discuss his or her epilepsy with a prospective employer.

Can someone not declare their epilepsy to an employer?

In the UK there is a legal requirement to answer truthfully all questions asked by an employer, including questions about medical conditions. Employers need this medical information to ensure that they are fulfilling the requirements of the Health and Safety at Work Act. If they are not informed and they then find out, the employee could be dismissed without recourse to an industrial tribunal.

Useful things to know

● No special insurance is needed for a worker with epilepsy as employer's liability insurance covers everyone in the workplace, including people with epilepsy or any kind of disability, provided that the employer is aware of the disability before the applicant accepted the job.

● It is the policy of the Occupational Pensions Board that if someone is fit enough to be employed, they are eligible for the pension scheme if one exists.

● The TUC and virtually all trade unions have positive policies on the employment of people with disabilities. Where there are allegations of discrimination at work because of epilepsy, the trade union should be able to help. Advice can also be sought from the Citizens Advice Bureau and from epilepsy organizations.

● Machinery in the workplace should have safety guards in place to comply with safety regulations protecting all workers as anyone could faint or slip while using it. If a special guard is required, subsidies are obtainable from the employment service (via the DEA).

Driving

Enquiries about driving regulations regarding epilepsy are among the most common. It is important to know what the law states, and this may differ from country to country. In the UK the driving regulations for people with epilepsy are as follows:

● A driving licence will be issued provided that all normal requirements are fulfilled and the applicant has been completely free of seizures for one year; or

● A licence will be given to someone who continues to have seizures provided that they happen only when the person is asleep. This pattern has to have been established over a three-year period.

Of course, no applicants must be likely to be a source of danger to the public.

When someone with epilepsy wants to

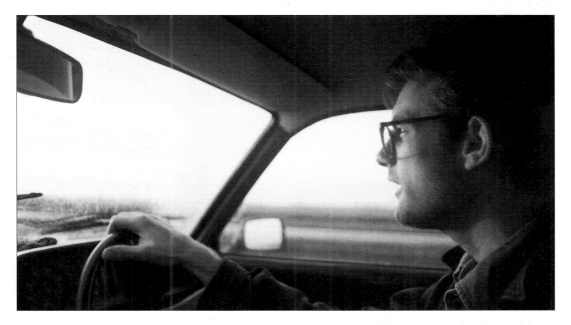

Having had no seizures for one year, people with epilepsy can reapply for their driving licence.

Living with epilepsy

drive for the first time, they should complete the standard application form. They will then be sent another form asking for details about their epilepsy and their doctor will also be asked to provide information.

If someone who already has a driving licence is diagnosed as having epilepsy, they must stop driving and must notify the Driving and Vehicle Licensing Authority (DVLA) in Swansea. The situation should be discussed fully with the doctor who will inform the individual of the legal situation. However, it is not up to the doctor to inform the DVLA; it is the responsibility of the person holding the driving licence. Anyone who continues to drive once the diagnosis of epilepsy has been made is driving illegally until the driving regulations set out above have been complied with. If someone drives illegally, their motor insurance is invalid and they are committing a criminal offence. When someone has fulfilled the above requirements they can then reapply to the DVLA which will request more medical information. Driving regulations can change, so it is important to make sure that you are up to date.

For the driver, what is meant by seizures?

From a driving point of view, seizures include all types of seizure, even those during which consciousness is not lost.

What about LGV and PCV licences?

To be able to hold a large goods vehicle (LGV) or passenger carrying vehicle (PCV) licence an individual 'must not have a continuing liability to seizures'. This means that they must have had no seizures or treatment for seizures for at least ten years and also have no neurological evidence of a continuing liability to seizures. These regulations also apply if a full licence rather than a renewable three-year licence is required.

What if any changes are made to my anti-epileptic medication?

Usually, if someone's anti-epileptic medication is being changed, it is advised that they stop driving for a period of six months, although there are no legal regulations surrounding this issue.

Making an appeal

In the UK the DVLA decision to withdraw a driving licence can be contested by lodging an appeal at a magistrate's court in England and Wales, or a sheriff's court in Scotland, within 30 days of the decision to withdraw the licence being notified in writing to the licence holder. More information on the appeal procedure is available from the DVLA, and again contacting an epilepsy organization will provide an opportunity to discuss the situation.

Motor insurance

Some motor insurance companies weight insurance premiums heavily against people with a history of epilepsy. Some will refuse to provide insurance at all. There are companies, however, which do give fair quotations and it is important to contact as many as possible to find the best cover. Epilepsy organizations often have information regarding insurance companies about which people with epilepsy have given favourable reports.

Transport

Rail travel

In the UK people with epilepsy who still have seizures despite treatment may apply for the Disabled Person's Railcard which gives discounts on many British Rail services. Application forms are available from main BR stations and should be accompanied by a letter from the applicant's registered medical practitioner.

Bus travel

In some areas people who cannot drive because of their epilepsy can get bus passes giving discounts on bus travel. This does vary from area to area as there is no national scheme in place. It is worthwhile checking with the local bus station.

Leisure time

How people spend their leisure time is important, not only for their physical well-being but also for a healthy state of mind. People who are continuing to have seizures need to think carefully about how to minimize any risks involved in taking part in potentially hazardous leisure activities. Parents of a child with active epilepsy will need to talk to the child's teachers about ways of enabling him or her to do activities like swimming and adventure outings while making sure that appropriate precautions are taken where necessary. People who have total control of

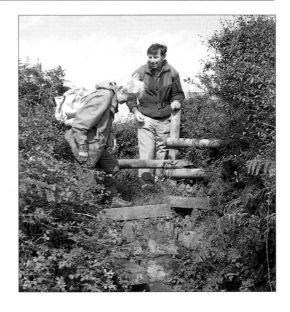

Keeping healthy and active is vital for everyone, including people with epilepsy.

Living with epilepsy

their seizures and have had for some time will not need to take the same precautions as those who still have seizures. This is also true for people who have only simple partial seizures when they do not lose consciousness and for those who have seizures only during their sleep. Since living a full and active life is so important for everyone, let's look at what can be done to make some of these leisure activities safer for people with active epilepsy.

Swimming

As long as there is someone either in the water or at the pool side who knows that there is a possibility that the swimmer may have a seizure in the water and who knows what to do

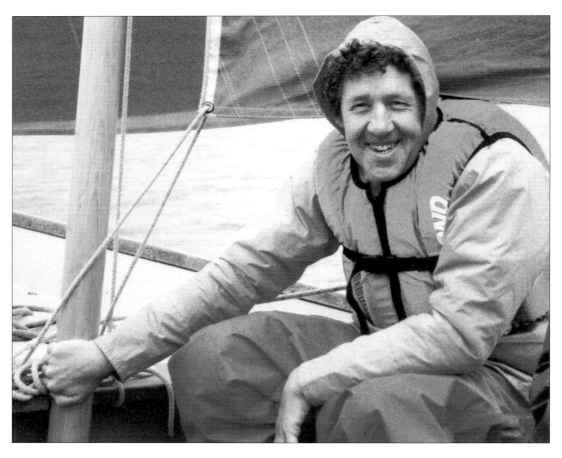

Sports such as sailing and canoeing need not be ruled out provided that there is adequate supervision.

should this happen, risks involved in swimming are minimal. The life guard at the pool should always be told if a swimmer with epilepsy is present. If someone has a tonic clonic seizure in the water, their head needs to be held above the surface while the seizure lasts and they should be taken from the water once it is over.

Water sports

Sailing, canoeing and windsurfing also need not be ruled out provided that there is someone on hand to manage the seizure if necessary. Other more dangerous water sports, such as sub aqua diving, involve much greater risks and are not advised.

Climbing and riding

It is advisable to do sports such as climbing and riding under appropriate guidance from experts who can provide the help needed should a seizure occur. Of course, the appropriate safety headgear should be worn at all times. It may be necessary to contact one of the organizations listed on page 79 to find out where such supervised activities can be done.

Travelling abroad

People with epilepsy who travel by air are advised to inform the cabin crew if they are likely to have a seizure. Flying does not itself trigger seizures, but if someone is very anxious, excited or becomes overtired as a result of jet lag, this may prove a problem.

Obtaining travel insurance is not usually difficult.

All medication should be carried in hand luggage in case suitcases are mislaid during the journey. It is often useful to keep anti-epileptic medication in its original container and to have duplicates of a letter from the family doctor stating the medical condition and the medication prescribed for it. These may be requested at international borders, particularly when crossing the borders of countries in the developing world. Taking adequate supplies of medication to cover the time away is vital unless using a company which will send medication to the requested destination. Another alternative would be to obtain the medication while abroad; however, it is important to be aware that in other countries some anti-epileptic drugs are known under different names or sometimes not available at all.

Safety in the home

Everyone should be aware of the importance of safety in the home. However, if someone has epilepsy which is not well controlled by medication, extra care needs to be taken, particularly if their seizures involve a sudden loss of consciousness with little or no warning.

Living with epilepsy

Let us consider safety around the house.

Kitchen

● If possible, use a microwave rather than a conventional oven.

● Use plastic microwavable containers instead of glass dishes.

● If you have to use a conventional oven, consider using the back rings or burners rather than those at the front and turn pan handles away to minimize the risk of someone falling and knocking the pan over.

● Grill food rather than frying it as this can be less dangerous.

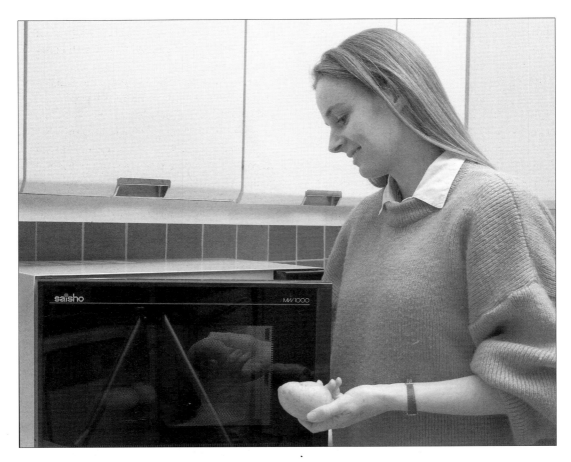

Safety in the home is important for everyone, especially for those with uncontrolled epilepsy. Microwave cooking is far safer than using a conventional oven.

74

● Use cordless irons and automatic cordless jug kettles with a safety lid and safety cut-out.

● Use trolleys to transfer from the oven to the table food and hot dishes which might cause injury if someone were to fall while carrying them.

● Buy items such as sauces in plastic rather than glass bottles.

● Use non-slip scatter carpets, rugs or carpet tiles in places where food may be spilt as they are cheaper to replace than fitted carpets.

Bathroom

For people with uncontrolled epilepsy having a shower is far more advisable than taking a bath; even so, if possible, showers with high-sided bases should be avoided as they could trap water if the drain were covered. If someone with epilepsy has to use a bath rather than a shower, the following points are worth considering:

● Shallow baths are safer than full baths.

● Have a bath only when there is someone else in the house who could help if necessary and make sure they know that you are having a bath.

● An 'Engaged' sign on an unlocked door allows privacy but means that access can be gained in case of emergency.

● Run the cold water before the hot water and turn the taps off before getting into the bath.

Bedroom

Some people who have nocturnal seizures prefer to use safety pillows and these are available from Helpful Hands at the address listed on page 79. For most people with epilepsy, however, it will not be necessary to take such precautions. Smoking in bed is never to be recommended, particularly for people with uncontrolled epilepsy.

Furniture

When choosing carpets and upholstery, care should be taken to avoid coarse fabrics which could result in friction burns and also fabrics which are difficult to clean. Fireproof fabrics and furniture are widely available and should be seriously considered by people with epilepsy who smoke.

If possible, enclose hot pipes and consider using radiator guards to prevent burns if someone falls against them. Try to avoid light free-standing heaters which could easily be knocked over in a seizure; for open or metal-cased fires a fire guard secured to the floor or wall is important. Turning the hot water thermostat down by a few degrees means that the water is never scalding hot.

Using safety glass in both doors and low windows greatly minimizes injury if someone falls against them, but safety film is also available which, when applied to door or window glass, prevents splintering. Bathroom and lavatory doors should preferably be hung so that they open outwards to prevent them being blocked by a person falling behind them. Avoiding the use of locks or using safety locks which can be operated from the outside is advisable.

There should always be an adequate number of electric sockets to avoid the danger of trailing flexes. Make sure that household insurance cover is good as seizure-related accidents can be expensive.

Living with epilepsy

Storing medication safely

Great care needs to be taken to store medication safely, particularly with children around. Anti-epileptic and other drugs should be locked away unless they need to be carried with you. Keeping anti-epileptic medication in a drug wallet (see page 42) prevents medication being taken twice and means that the original containers can be stored out of the reach of children.

Safety outside the home

People with uncontrolled epilepsy may want to wear or carry with them something which states that they have epilepsy. This idea does not appeal to everyone, but for those to whom it does there are several options available.

Bracelets and necklaces are available from the Medic-Alert Foundation and also from SOS Talisman (see page 79 for addresses). Most epilepsy organizations produce information cards which can hold personal details, information on what type of seizures the bearer has, what medication they are taking and what bystanders should do if they have a seizure.

Safety is an important consideration for everyone. People with uncontrolled epilepsy need to take extra care, but it is important not to go to unnecessary extremes. Everyone takes risks on a day-to-day basis, and while it is sensible to eliminate unnecessary risks, it is vitally important to live a full and active life and not to be constantly thinking of potential hazards.

The National Society for Epilepsy (NSE)

There is a number of national epilepsy organizations but the NSE, as well as being one of the largest, is one of the oldest, having provided epilepsy services for over 100 years. Today the NSE is one of the most well-known centres of expertise in the world, offering a range of services for people with epilepsy, including:

- an MR scanning unit dedicated to epilepsy;
- short-term medical assessment;
- longer-term residential care;
- respite care;
- information and education;
- rehabilitation;
- outpatient services;
- a community network of self-help groups;
- associate membership.

Chapter seven

Looking forward to conquering epilepsy

There is still a great deal about the workings of the human brain which we do not understand. However, advancements in brain scanning and research techniques are providing scientists and doctors with greater insight into how the brain works and – importantly when looking at conditions like epilepsy – why it sometimes doesn't work as it should. Research is also being done into possible genetic causes, bringing hope that one day those genetic faults responsible for causing some forms of epilepsy can eventually be corrected.

Epilepsy surgery is increasingly becoming a realistic option for greater numbers of people, and as surgical and scanning techniques improve the risks involved with this type of treatment will become minimal and the already high success rate will rise even higher. Other forms of treatment are also being researched (vagus nerve stimulation being the newest of alternative surgical treatments), and as more people become interested in alternative or complementary therapies such as biofeedback, breakthroughs in these areas could be imminent.

New forms of anti-epileptic medications are constantly being tested and developed, and as more of these reach the open market the number of drugs from which doctors can choose to treat their patients will increase. It is hoped that the future will bring anti-epileptic drugs with few or no side effects and that doctors will be able to select exactly the right drug to control their patient's seizures first time round.

Perhaps the most important advancement, however, has been made in the field of educating the general public about epilepsy. Not so many years ago very little was known or understood about, for instance, cancer, Parkinson's disease or Aids, and because there was ignorance there was also fear. Good education programmes have meant that these illnesses are now spoken about openly, are generally understood and are accepted in our society, and this in turn has made life easier for people living with these medical conditions. People with epilepsy deserve that same understanding which can only come when the myths, stigma and misconceptions which still surround the condition have been broken down by improved knowledge and a greater awareness of what epilepsy is, and in this we can all play a part.

Together we can look forward to conquering epilepsy.

Looking forward to conquering epilepsy

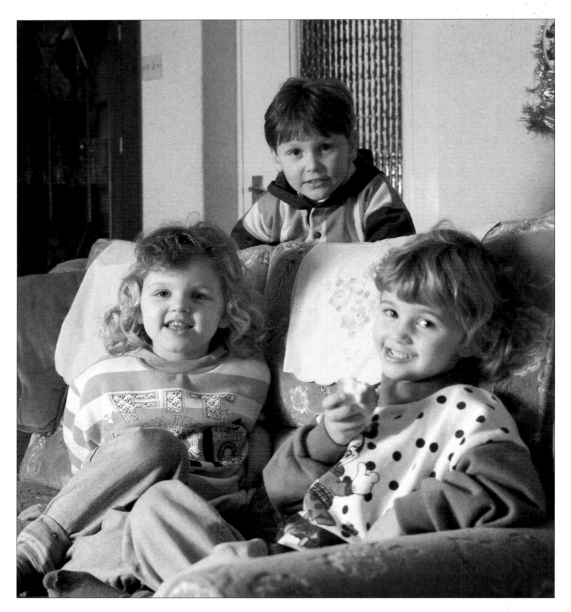

Advancement is constantly being made in treatments for epilepsy and so we can look forward to the future positively.

Useful addresses

The National Society for Epilepsy (NSE)

Keeping up to date with the latest developments is important and you can do this by joining the NSE as an associate member. The society will also advise you regarding regional groups and associations. Details are available from the address below.

The National Society for Epilepsy
Chalfont St Peter
Gerrards Cross
Buckinghamshire SL9 0RJ
Tel: (including helpline) 01494 873991

British Epilepsy Association
Tel: (helpline) 0800 309030

British Herbal Medicine
PO Box 304
Bournemouth
Dorset BH7 6JZ

British Homeopathic Association
27a Devonshire Street
London W1N 1RJ

British Holistic Medical Association
179 Gloucester Place
London NW1 6DX

British Sports Association for the Disabled
Tel: 0171 490 4919

Centre for Advice on Natural Alternatives
Tyddyn y Mynydd
Waullapria
Llanelly Hill
Abergavenny
Gwent WP7 0PN

Disabled Living Foundation
Tel: 0171 289 6111
Provides an information service about aids and facilities

Driving Vehicle Licensing Authority (DVLA)
Tel: 01792 782341

DSS Benefit Enquiry Line
Tel: 0800 666555

Epilepsy Bereaved
PO Box 1777
Bournemouth
Dorset BH5 1YR
Offers support to families and friends

Helpful Hands
2 Chester Road
Macclesfield
Cheshire SK10 1AU
Tel: 01625 617857

Jubilee Sailing Trust
Tel: 01703 631 388

Medic-Alert Foundation
12 Bridge Wharf
156 Caledonian Road
London N1 9UU
Tel: 0171 833 3034

NHS Epilepsy Assessment Units

The National Society for Epilepsy
Address as above left

Bootham Park Hospital
Bootham
York YO3 7BY
Tel: 01904 610777

Park Hospital for Children
Old Road
Headington
Oxford OX3 7LQ
Tel: 01865 741717

Riding for the Disabled
Tel: 01203 696510

Royal Association for Disability and Rehabilitation (RADAR)
Tel: 0171 250 3222
Offers information, advice and support

SOS Talisman
Talman Ltd
21 Grays Court
Ley Street
Ilford
Essex IG2 7RQ
Tel: 0181 554 5579

Australia

National Epilepsy Association of Australia
PO BOX 554
Lilydale
Victoria 3140
Australia

USA

Epilepsy Foundation of America
4351 Garden City Drive
Landover
Maryland 20785
USA

Index